D0906041

WEIGHT TRAINING
IN ATHLETICS
AND
PHYSICAL EDUCATION

WEIGHT TRAINING
IN ATHLETICS
AND
PHYSICAL EDUCATION

GENE HOOKS
Director of Athletics
Wake Forest University

Prentice-Hall, Inc., *Englewood Cliffs, New Jersey*

Library of Congress Cataloging in Publication Data

Hooks, Gene.
  Weight training in athletics and physical education.

  Includes bibliographies.
  1. Weight lifting. 2. Muscle strength. I. Title
[DNLM: 1. Physical education and training.
2. Sports. QT255 H78w 1974]
GV546.H66   796.4'1   74-592
ISBN 0-13-947994-5

10   9

Prentice-Hall International, Inc., *London*
Prentice-Hall of Australia, Pty, Ltd., *Sydney*
Prentice-Hall of Canada, Ltd., *Toronto*
Prentice-Hall of India Private Limited, *New Delhi*
Prentice-Hall of Japan, Inc., *Tokyo*

Dedicated to my wife
Jean
and to our boys
Dave, Denny, and Mike

CONTENTS

PREFACE

The idea that an athlete should train with weights is based on the assumption that strength is the key to athletic success, and that weight training is the best way to develop strength. Weights have been lifted for many purposes and in every conceivable way. The author does not claim originality in developing a drastically new program of weight training. The programs presented are not intended to be revolutionary. They result from years of research and study of the training programs of many experts, experimentation with many athletes, and interviews with players, coaches, physical educators, team trainers, and physicians. They have been tried and proved by college athletic squads.

There is a right way and a wrong way to train with weights, depending entirely on one's objectives. The primary aim of this book is to apply weight training to athletic programs. Step-by-step training programs are presented for many sports, incorporating weight training into each.

Other portions of the book are written for those persons who wish to weight-train with other objectives in mind. One chapter is devoted to the use of weights in physical education classes. Another part is written on the prevention and rehabilitation of certain injuries. Another is on fitness. And another is on competitive lifting. Each of these weight training programs differ according to the objectives of the lifters.

The material is so arranged that a coach or player interested only in training for one sport need not read the entire book. He can begin a program by reading only the chapter dealing with the sport in which he is interested. However, in order to get the full benefit of the book he should also read the first five chapters, which will provide him with the background material he needs to conduct a sound program. The same general chapter outline is followed for each of the sports to make the presentation more simple and the material easier to find.

The exercises and drills described throughout the book are numbered consecutively. To facilitate their use, the number of the drill is included in parentheses beside the particular drill each time that drill is listed. A list of drills is also included.

I am deeply indebted to the many people who have helped make this book a reality. Those who read portions of the original manuscript and offered suggestions for its improvement were: Russell Brantley, Wake Forest University News Bureau; Dr. Robert Prichard, Bowman Gray School of Medicine, Wake Forest University; and former Wake Forest coaches Jack Stallings (baseball), Jack Murdock and Horace McKinney (basketball), Bill Hildebrand (football), Bill Jordan (track), and Leo Ellison (swimming). In the revised addition the present coaching staff has been most helpful.

Special words of thanks are extended to my wife, Jean, who did the excellent drawings, assisted in preparing the manuscript, and bore with me throughout; and to Mrs. Rebecca Waggoner, who rendered expert and faithful assistance as typist and proofreader for this edition.

G. Hooks

WEIGHT TRAINING
IN ATHLETICS
AND
PHYSICAL EDUCATION

1

STRENGTH,

THE FORGOTTEN KEY

Strength is the key to success in modern athletics. Such a statement may sound extreme, but nevertheless it is true. The coach who capitalizes on this knowledge is destined for success. The coach who doesn't is destined for mediocrity. This book is written in the belief that the importance of strength has been and is being overlooked by far too many coaches and players. A sound mind and a sound body are man's most precious possessions. In most sports the athlete must have this foundation upon which to build. There are, however, many special elements needed for athletic success. Probably the four basic ones are coordination, desire, speed, and strength. As a rule, the majority of a coach's time is devoted to teaching coordination in the individual skills and techniques, the fundamentals of the sport. The other three are recognized but usually passed over hurriedly as inherent elements that cannot be greatly influenced. This may be true for desire, and to some extent speed, but it is in no way true for strength. There is a great deal that can and should be done to make an athlete stronger. Any athlete can improve his strength, and with it his overall performance. A good coach will exploit this knowledge to win many extra contests.

There is a vast need for everyone involved in athletics to better understand strength. There are two very good reasons why this element of athletic success should be studied carefully, especially by coaches. First, they must realize that they are today working with a weaker athlete. The mechanization of modern life has robbed our youth of the many manual chores that once developed strong bodies. Unless something is done to change our way of life, future athletes will be increasingly weak.

Secondly, coaches must realize that improved strength will *help* an athlete, not hurt him. Strength has long been swaddled in ignorance and superstition.

Most coaches recognize it as a valuable asset to athletic success, but few know how to use it to advantage. When a big, strong boy happens along, the average coach will eagerly teach him the skill and technique he needs to be a good athlete. The same coach might not dare develop strength in a highly skilled athlete, even though strength is much easier to improve than technique.

Strength in athletes must be studied just as one would study technique, speed, and desire. All four elements are valuable and need special attention. Strength, however, is the key element because it is more easily improved than the others. It is, in fact, the one element that can be improved with one hundred percent success.

THE AGE OF PUSH BUTTONS

The American people are gradually degenerating. Man needs vigorous exercise in order to grow and develop. Muscle must be overloaded in order to be strengthened. If it is adequately overloaded it grows in size and strength. If not, it weakens and degenerates. That is exactly what is happening to us, because ours is a generation of inactivity.

In recent years we have been provided with countless labor-saving devices. Television sets have become standard furniture in every home. In this age of mechanization, work weeks have been and will continue to be shortened. Most families have one automobile, and many have two. So completely has our society been mechanized that some economists predict the near extinction of the man who works with his hands within ten to twelve years.

This age of inactivity apparently knows no age limits. The activity of the average family pivots around the availability of the family automobile. A father's most vigorous activity during a typical day is getting in the car and driving to work. With the family car available there is little need for the children to walk or to ride a bicycle. Even if they wanted to they would probably find in place of their favorite paths networks of highways with steady streams of traffic. There is no wood to cut or coal to carry. There are many lawns to mow, but one has only to follow a power mower. In fact, the average young boy growing up in America doesn't have an opportunity to perform manual labor, even if he so desires.

A study sponsored by the American Association for Health, Physical Education, and Recreation compared the physical fitness of American youths with that of youths from England, Scotland, Wales, and Cyprus. Our young people were found to be as much as 14 percent below those of the other countries for all tests and at all ages between 10 and 17 years. On the arm-strength test the British were, on the average, 19 percent better.[1] This report is very similar to earlier comparisons with the youth of Japan and some European countries. These reports don't necessarily reflect on our youth,

[1] *Winston-Salem Journal,* December 7, 1960, p. 1.

because they were probably no different from the others at birth. It is a reflection, however, on our way of life. We have robbed our youth of the opportunity to develop normally.

Today only a small percentage of the American people are participating regularly in some form of athletics. By far the larger majority are casually observing. Most of us satisfy our athletic inclinations by watching a highly skilled group of athletes play on television. The more hardy spectators drive to the stadiums or gymnasiums to get a closer look.

Physical activity is certainly not a part of our way of life. Of the small percentage of participation, much is confined to school and college physical education and intramural programs. A small group of the most talented play in competitive athletic programs. The two most popular sports for the post-school group are golf and bowling. These are interesting and enjoyable games, but they probably owe their popularity to the fact that they are *not* particularly strenuous. The exercise that once was available in golf is being rapidly removed by electric carts. Is it not a sad commentary on the American way of life that those who participate in these sports are looked on as our physically *most* active citizens?

The degeneration of Americans had become such a problem that former President Eisenhower created a Council on Youth Fitness (at the cabinet level) and appointed a Citizens Advisory Committee on Fitness of American Youth. This emphasis certainly didn't halt the degeneration. Physical fitness tests in some colleges continued to show a steady decline in the strength of freshmen.

President Kennedy took steps to provide the leadership for a vigorous fitness program. That such an action was necessary is alarming. That the United States had leadership which recognized the problem and took steps to halt the deterioration of our people was encouraging. The basic steps were as follows:

1. Kennedy appointed a White House Committee on Health and Fitness to formulate and carry out a program to improve the physical condition of the nation.
2. He made the physical fitness of our youth the direct responsibility of the Department of Health, Education and Welfare. This department was to conduct research into the development of a physical fitness program for the nation's public schools.
3. The governor of each state was to be invited to attend an annual National Youth Fitness Congress to examine the progress that had been made in physical fitness during the preceding years and exchange suggestions for improvement.
4. The president and all departments of government made it clear that the promotion of sports participation and physical fitness was a basic, continuing policy of the United States.[2]

[2]John F. Kennedy, "The Soft American," *Sports Illustrated,* December 26, 1960, p. 17.

Successive administrations have continued to support the initiative of Presidents Eisenhower and Kennedy. President Nixon has enthusiastically supported fitness and sports programs at all levels. However, the results are not encouraging and the coach of modern athletic teams should be acutely aware of the degeneration of the American people; he should also recognize that the material he inherits will be increasingly weak, though it may not be apparent. Those coaches who take steps to prevent or correct such an occurrence will have a tremendous advantage over their opponents.

STRENGTH IN ATHLETICS

The value of strength in athletics is not a new idea by any means. The fact that high school and college coaches have accepted its importance has been reflected in their teams for years. Agreement is almost unanimous that "the good big man will always beat the good little man." The statement would be even more true if it read, "the good strong man will always beat the good weak man."

One has only to look at the size and strength of the outstanding teams in the world today to realize the value of strength in athletics. Very seldom does a lineman in professional football weigh less than 225 pounds, or a back less than 200 pounds. In professional basketball the skinny player is a thing of the past, and in college basketball he is at a terrific disadvantage. Professional baseball players are not as big as football and basketball players, but they are certainly bigger and much stronger than the average man. The same is true in other sports. These players are big not just in bulk, but in muscle. They are successful because they are highly skilled, but when players of equal skill meet, the stronger one has a tremendous advantage.

So many times we have heard a coach shrug off a losing season with "you can't win without the horses." And it's generally true that no matter how much a coach may do to improve technique and strategy, his record will be only as good as his material. Granted one coach will occasionally out-mastermind the other, but this will ordinarily occur when two teams are evenly matched. Very few coaches know so much more about a sport than their associates that they can win in spite of mediocre material.

The most successful coaches are those with enough foresight to ensure a steady flow of good material. In high schools this flow is usually accomplished by organizing the sport in junior high and grammar school grades, and by teaching the skills and techniques of the game to everyone. An occasional lean year is experienced, but the players are usually highly skilled and the teams highly successful. In future years, however, a feeder program of this type will not get the job done unless something is also done about the basic body strength of these youngsters.

The more popular sports demand strength for success, but by their nature do little to develop it. In order to develop the arms and shoulders the muscles in these areas must be overloaded. If a boy plays baseball he handles nothing heavier than a thirty-three ounce bat. A golf club, a tennis racket, and a basketball are even lighter. There is very little muscular development in the arms and shoulders to be gained by participating in any of these activities. The legs are adequately strengthened, but without some hard physical labor to develop his arms a boy will be mediocre in most any athletic activity. The data collected so far indicate conclusively that the best athletes are stronger in the arms and shoulders, and further, that strength in this body area is generally an indication of potential athletic excellence.

STRENGTH IS THE KEY

For many years the philosophy of high school coaches as well as college and professional recruiters and coaches has been to seek out the stronger boys in hopes that they can be taught the proper techniques and skills of the desired sport. This policy has become increasingly apparent in recent years as the strength of our youth has deteriorated. By all means the talents of the stronger boys should continue to be developed to the fullest. They usually turn out to be outstanding athletes. But isn't it about time we stopped neglecting the individual who is skilled but who is too small and weak to play in good competition? It has been pointed out that improvement in sport technique requires a certain amount of natural ability. Improvement in strength requires only short bouts of hard work administered with some degree of common sense. Why not devise programs to improve the strength and power of the boys who lack basic body strength? Many of them will develop into the very best athletes.

The best way to develop strength is through an organized program of weight training. Today only a small number of coaches are using weights on an organized basis to supplement their athletic programs. Some conveniently ignore weight training because they have heard that it will make one stiff and tight; that it will cause one to lose his touch; that it will make one musclebound; or that the boys will want to become "Atlases" and forget about athletics. The good coach can eliminate all these criticisms if he conducts a sensible training program.

To be successful, the high school coach must make the same effort to promote strength-building in the school system that he makes to promote the junior high and junior varsity athletic programs. It takes much more than one set of weights in the corner of the gym and a lot of lip service about the program at the touchdown club. It must be made an integral part of his feeder program, not for just a few of the more promising players, but for any and all boys he can interest. Strength and power are accessible to all. If the program is started during junior high school while the body is developing and maturing rapidly and is continued through high school, many boys will be successful who otherwise would never have been given a chance. For the same reason, college coaches should start the strength-building program for their freshmen teams at the earliest possible date.

College coaches should recruit with the knowledge that strength can be readily developed through weight training. If a boy is outstanding in high school simply because he is stronger than everyone else, he may have a very difficult time in college. Speed, skill, and desire are much more important qualities to look for. If a boy has these, he has a chance to be outstanding, even if he is relatively weak, when he attends college. All he needs is the desire to be the best. The necessary strength can be added through weight training to make such a boy as good as he wants to be.

Whether he is in a high school or a college, the coach's job is not only to provide the opportunity but also to provide the leadership, the supervision, and the motivation to develop each player to his maximum ability. Many outstanding coaches have accepted this truth and are conducting organized weight-training programs for their squads. Others must follow their lead if they hope to compete on equal terms.

2

MUSCLE

The coach who embarks on a program of weight training has two immediate problems. First, he must design a program of training that will be applicable to his immediate situation. Second, he must sell the program to his players and to the school administrators.

Weight-training programs outlined in this book are applicable to many situations, but to design enough programs to fit the needs of all prevailing situations would be impossible. Many factors influence the program and must be considered individually. Facilities and equipment are considered first, of course, but all too often these factors determine the entire nature and scope of the program. To conduct a sound program and to interpret it properly to the players, the parents, and the administration, the more basic factors must be considered by the coach. What is muscle? What are its characteristics? How does it cause movement? What causes it to contract? What are its limits? How does it grow in strength and size? What about endurance and fatigue? What is the effect of weight training on muscle?

No pretense is made that all of these questions are answered in this chapter. Many are, but a complete coverage of muscle is far beyond the scope of this book. A basic knowledge is imperative, however, and any coach would do well to explore the workings of muscles and examine his coaching technique and philosophy in the light of this knowledge. A brief overview of the strength, the structure, and the function of muscle is presented in this chapter. It is hoped it will be used as an aid in better understanding weight training and properly interpreting the program to all parties concerned.

ANATOMY AND PHYSIOLOGY OF MUSCLE

There are over 400 skeletal muscles, which make up from 40 to 50 percent of the body's total weight. The function of these muscles is the production of movements and maintenance of posture, and in so doing, is responsible for such activities as walking, talking, breathing, chewing, swallowing, playing sports, and countless others.

Skeletal muscles are closely related to other body systems. They are dependent on the respiratory, digestive, and circulatory systems for energy and nourishment; on the excretory system for elimination of wastes; on the skin for protection; and on the nervous system for the stimulus to contract. In turn these systems depend on the muscles for locomotion and other previously listed movements and functions.

A muscle, by definition, is a bundle of contractile fibers encased in a sheath of connective tissue. The fibers are elongated and cylindrical and each is enclosed in a thin elastic membrane much like a link of sausage. Units of 100 to 150 fibers are bound into bundles, and these bundles are in turn held together in larger bundles. The entire muscle is enclosed in a membrane, or sheath. The various sheaths merge at the ends to form tendons which in turn attach the muscles to the bone. The end of the muscle that is attached to the stationary part of the skeleton is termed the origin, while the end attached to the movable part of the skeleton is termed the insertion. The origin is usually a fleshy attachment to the bone, while the insertion is attached to the bone by means of a tendon. The muscle pulls from the origin and the insertion toward the center, or the belly, of the muscle.

The number of muscle fibers varies according to the size and function of the muscle. The arrangement of fibers within the muscle also varies. They are generally arranged longitudinally with the long axis of the muscle; but they may curve, converge to a common tendon, or take more complex shapes. These shapes are important because the longitudinal direction of the fiber determines the direction of pull on the bones, because the fibers always contract from the end to the middle.

The thickness and strength of the connective tissues vary a great deal, depending upon the location and strength of the muscle. If the muscle is connected to the bone in an exposed area such as the knee or ankle, the connective tissue is very heavy, to give additional protection. In a well-protected muscle deep within the body, the connective tissue is less prevalent. The thickness of the connective tissue also varies with the body condition; thin in weak, soft muscles, thick and tough in strong, hard muscles.

Blood Circulation in Muscle

Oxygen, sugar and other foodstuffs for the muscles are delivered by the circulatory system. Arteries carry the blood from the heart. The arteries divide as they get farther from the heart into arterioles, which in turn divide into small capillaries. The muscle fibers are surrounded by a fantastic number of these tiny capillaries. The walls of the capillaries are thin and allow for easy passage of needed oxygen and foodstuffs to the fiber. Waste products are formed very rapidly in the muscles during exercise, bringing about a corresponding increase in the demand for oxygen and foodstuffs. The exchange of materials is facilitated by an increase in the flow of blood and lymph through the muscles. Waste products are carried away from the muscle by venules, which converge into larger veins as they get closer to the heart.

During free exercise the alternate contraction and relaxation of the muscles exerts a strong pumping action on the blood flow. When a muscle relaxes, the veins of that muscle become filled with blood. During contraction blood is squeezed out of the veins and forced back toward the heart. Valves in the veins prevent the blood from backing up. Obese tissue (fat) doesn't provide such assistance to the heart. Instead of acting as a booster pump as muscle does, it puts a drag on the entire circulatory system.

Physical Properties of Muscle

In some respects a muscle is like a rubber band. It can be stretched, and when the force causing the stretch is removed it will return to its original length. The lengthening property is referred to as extensibility, and the return to normal is called elasticity. Muscle, however, is much more versatile than a rubber band. It can shorten itself from its resting length by pulling both ends toward the belly. When the length of the muscle decreases in this manner, the circumference increases. This property of contractility is observed in the contraction of the biceps of the arm. Another characteristic property is viscosity. This is a resistance to a change in shape of the muscle, and is often referred to as the protective mechanism of the muscle. The muscular contraction is actually resisted slightly to lessen the likelihood of injury in sudden violent activity.

Movement

In normal physical activity a muscle contracts when stimulated by impulses brought to it by the motor nerves. Muscles move the various parts of the body by acting on the skeleton at the joints, or articulations. The bones function as levers while the joints function as their fulcrums. When a muscle contracts, it pulls on the two bones to which it is attached. If one of the bones is not anchored or stabilized, both of the bones will move toward the center. However, because one of the bones is usually anchored at the origin of the muscle, the movement will take place in the other bone, which is attached to the insertion end of the muscle. Therefore, when a muscle contracts it applies a force at the insertion end, and movement results. This is the general rule,

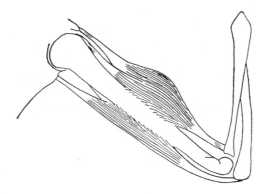

Figure 1. Arm flexion

although it is not unusual for the origin and the insertion to interchange if the insertion of the muscle is stabilized.

Movement is brought about by a coordinated action of muscle groups. Some muscles contract while others relax. Movement invariably involves two sets of muscles, which more or less act in opposition to one another. The group that contracts and furnishes the power is identified as the mover; the relaxing group is referred to as the antagonist. For example, if you wish to flex the arm, the biceps brachii (the mover) contracts, while the triceps brachii on the posterior portion of the arm (the antagonist) relaxes.

If you desire to return the arm to an extended or straight position the triceps brachii becomes the mover and contracts while the biceps brachii relaxes and becomes the antagonist. If the biceps brachii and the triceps brachii were contracted together, there would be no movement at the elbow joint; the arm would be locked in a straight position.

Movement thus results from the pulling action of certain muscles. In any strength-building program it is important to remember that a muscle always pulls and never pushes. Antagonist muscles will relax in varying degrees in order to steady movements, and in some situations will undergo lengthening contraction when the joint needs such protection, but they will not push. Antagonist muscles aid by relaxing, not pushing.

Muscle Tone

Muscles are under a slight degree of tension even when they are not being exerted. This results in a firmness of muscle and is referred to as muscle tone, or tonus. Very active muscles are much more apt to exhibit good tone than those used less. Certain muscles can be strengthened by resistive exercise and are said to exhibit a high degree of tone. Others may weaken from disuse and are said to exhibit a low degree of tone.

It is possible for improved tone to result in a shortening of muscle. This fact is used to advantage in corrective exercise to correct posture faults. A muscle group on one side of a joint can be strengthened and shortened while its antagonistic group is stretched, resulting in a new joint position. It is important to note that this can happen in weight training also if the program doesn't maintain a balance of exercises, with some for the muscle groups controlling each side of the joints. There is absolutely no possibility that this shortening of muscle will occur in a well-balanced training program.

Contraction of Muscle

The contraction to a simple stimulus is called a muscle twitch. A study of the twitch reveals that it does not respond immediately to the stimulus. There is a fraction of a second between the application of the stimulus and the contraction, known as the latent period. The muscles reach their peak contraction almost immediately (contraction phase) and then gradually resume their former length (relaxation phase). In a rapid series of twitches the contractions become progressively stronger, a phenomenon known as *treppe.*

If a muscle contracts but the resistance is so great that it cannot shorten, the contraction is known as an isometric or static contraction. If the resistance can be overcome and the muscle shortens, it is referred to as an isotonic or dynamic contraction.

STRENGTH OF MUSCLE

Strength of muscle is usually defined as the amount of force that a muscle is capable of exerting, such as in pushing, pulling, gripping, or lifting. The force varies, the degree depending on any one combination of the following factors:

1. Speed of contraction
2. Duration of contraction
3. Resistance
4. Muscular size
5. Readiness
6. Metabolism

Speed and Duration of Contraction

A rapidly contracting muscle is said to evidence a loss of strength, probably because of the increasing viscosity of the muscle. On the other hand, a muscle contracting very slowly loses a large amount of energy, because it must maintain the force over a long period of time. The most advantageous contraction, therefore, is one of moderate speed. This type of contraction uses to advantage the momentum that is gained in a faster movement and minimizes the loss of energy experienced in a slowly contracting muscle. Weight-lifting exercises are generally performed at this moderate speed, where pure strength is the primary objective. However, if explosive power is the major objective it would appear wise to so condition the muscle through rapid contractions as well.

Resistance

The amount of tension a muscle must exert to overcome a resistance is the key to muscular development. A muscle which contracts against a resistance that demands exertion increases in strength. The degree of the increase depends on the amount of resistance. If the muscle is strengthened enough to overcome the resistance easily, then that resistance is no longer exerting the muscle, and there is little if any gain in strength. In order for the muscle to make further gains, the amount of resistance must be increased. This is known as the overload principle. There is some doubt as to how much a muscle should be overloaded. Most theories of strength development suggest that the muscle should be overloaded enough to cause a maximum contraction but not to the extent that the resistance must be overcome by nerve, or "guts." Others suggest that the muscle will increase in strength more rapidly if it contracts maximally with no restraint. We have had excellent results at Wake Forest by encouraging a maximum effort after the players have gone through a proper conditioning program.

It should be noted that a muscle can be overloaded for endurance as well as strength. For maximum gains in strength it is necessary to overload the muscle enough to cause a maximum contraction. However, a gain in strength does not necessarily indicate a corresponding gain in endurance. For endurance training it is necessary to increase considerably the number of times the muscle will contract against a resistance. In this method of overloading, a light resistance or weight is used, but the speed of the contractions is usually increased.

In order to train for both strength and endurance, a compromise between the two programs has been devised. The muscles to be exercised are overloaded to the extent that they can perform an exercise a number of times. (Eight seems to be most popular although it ranges from six to fifteen.) The last repetition should be close to a maximum contraction. Thus, muscles are overloaded for gains in strength and endurance.

Muscular Size

As a muscle grows in strength, it grows in size, or hypertrophies. As a muscle loses in strength, it loses in size, or atrophies. The strength of a muscle therefore, is roughly equal to its circumference, other factors being equal. There is a difference in the quality of muscle, however, that is not generally understood. Some body-builders have impressive-looking muscles that are not especially strong, while others may not have as large a muscle but may have a great deal of muscular strength. Two players of equal size and strength often begin identical weight programs at the same time yet derive far different results. Some boys develop rapidly, while others are painfully slow. Differences in build often account for disparity, but the major cause seems to be an inherent variance in muscle quality.

It has previously been stated that a muscle is formed by many small muscle fibers. As the degree of resistance is increased, apparently the number of fibers contracting is increased up to a maximum contraction. It therefore takes a maximum contraction to exercise all of the fibers. These fibers do not change in number. The increase in size of a muscle is brought about by an increase in the cross section of each fiber. An apparent increase in the amount of connective tissue and in the number of capillaries may account for some of the growth. It is possible that exercise brings some dormant fibers into play, the growth of which could account for much of the hypertrophy. However, the change in muscular size is not yet clearly understood and is the subject of continued research.

Readiness

Stretching the muscle before stimulation within limits increases the force of the contraction. Stretched muscles are tensed and are thus able to exert a greater force at the start of the stimulation. This is one of the reasons the baseball fielder waits in a crouched position or the sprinter takes a crouched starting position. A crouch stretches the extensor muscles of the legs, enabling them to exert a stronger force. This advantage plus the advantageous position of the levers enables these athletes to get a better jump or break.

Metabolism

An adequate oxygen and fuel supply enables the muscle to contract with more strength. When this supply is limited in some way the contractile force, or strength of a muscle, is seriously impaired. Vigorous exercises, usually accompanied by strength gains, will increase the supply of oxygen and fuel. There will be increased efficiency of the circulatory system, which delivers the supplies to the muscle. This is brought about partly by an increased power in the heart, now able to deliver more blood with fewer beats. The newly formed capillaries provide for a more rapid supply of oxygen and foodstuffs to the muscles and also enable the muscle to rid itself more rapidly of waste products. An increased supply of chemical buffers in the blood can manage larger quantities of the waste acids. The larger, stronger muscle, by its contracting action, improves circulation. It is true that these changes occur most rapidly as a result of those exercises that provide for endurance as well as strength building. However, strength of a muscular contraction is obviously influenced by the metabolic conditions present, and a significant increase in strength will probably be accompanied by an improvement in these metabolic conditions.

ENDURANCE OF MUSCLE

Muscular endurance is the capability of continuing activity under the pain of fatigue. This happens in athletics when the overload emphasis is placed on the number of repetitions instead of the resistance of each load. For example, you would develop the endurance of the biceps brachii by flexing the arm many times with a light weight.

The primary physiological adjustment evidenced in athletes with great endurance is the great increase in the number of capillaries in the muscles. There is also an increase in the efficiency of the heart to pump blood to the muscles. These two results enable the circulatory system to furnish the working muscles with an adequate supply of blood. This blood is rich in oxygen because of a more efficient ventilation of the lungs and is richer in glucose and other foodstuffs in a well-conditioned athlete.

Weight training as controlled by the circulatory and respiratory systems does not affect the endurance of an athlete significantly because it is not carried out continuously over a long enough period of time. Distance swimming and distance running develop cardio-respiratory endurance because they involve a prolonged rhythmical exercise of a large number of the body's muscles. Some athletes respond to endurance training more quickly than others. It is generally felt among coaches that it takes at least five or six weeks to develop enough endurance for most sports. After that length of time athletes should be in shape for competition.

Fatigue

Fatigue is evidenced by the diminished capacity of the muscles to contract or respond to a stimulus. The exact nature of fatigue is not known, but there is reason to believe that muscular fatigue is the loss of the individual's capacity to transmit nerve impulses from the brain and spinal cord to the muscle. There is probably a chemical factor involved, but this factor is not well understood. Fatigue operates as a safety precaution in that one's capacity for muscular exertion is directly related to his willingness to exert. Usually the loss of the will to exert precedes any physiological damage to the muscle. In order to postpone fatigue the trainee must learn to endure its pain, at least to the degree that he is conditioned to participate in his sport with no obvious discomfort.

SELECTED REFERENCES

Anthony, Catherine Parker, and Norma Jane Kolthoff, *Textbook of Anatomy and Physiology*, 8th ed. St. Louis: The C. V. Mosby Company, 1971.

Broer, Marion R., *Efficiency of Human Movement*, 2nd ed. Philadelphia: W. B. Saunders Company, 1966.

Karpovitch, Peter V., and Wayne E. Sinning, *Physiology of Muscular Activity*, 7th ed. Philadelphia: W. B. Saunders Company, 1971.

Morehouse, Laurence E., and Augustus T. Miller, *Physiology of Exercise*, 5th ed. St. Louis: The C. V. Mosby Company, 1967.

Murray, Jim, and Peter V. Karpovitch, *Weight Training in Athletics*. Englewood Cliffs, N.J.: Prentice-Hall, Inc., 1956.

Rasch, Philip J., and Roger K. Burke, *Kinesiology and Applied Anatomy*. Philadelphia: Lea & Febiger, 1971.

Wells, Katherine F., *Kinesiology*, 4th ed. Philadelphia: W. B. Saunders Company, 1966.

3

STRENGTH
DEVELOPMENT

The principle of any method of strength development is the same: the muscle has to be overloaded in order for the strength of the muscle to be increased. There are many methods by which this might be accomplished. Some of the more popular ones are: (1) calisthenics, (2) isometric contractions, (3) isometrics with weights, (4) isokinetics, (5) metal springs and rubber cables, and (6) weight lifting and/or weight training. The results of the various methods are not the same, however, because the intensity of the overloads on the muscle is much different, the methods of applying the overload are different, and the durations of the overloads are controlled differently. In spite of these differences, strength is improved with each method. In the final analysis the major difference in the application of the overload on the muscle rests with the attitude and zest of the exerciser, although there are several basic and inherent differences in the systems which influence appreciably the results that might be expected.

CALISTHENICS PROGRAM

Calisthenics programs are not always conducive to maximum strength gains. It is true that calisthenics such as push-ups, chins, sit-ups, and so forth, overload the participating muscles, thereby improving strength; but because of individual differences in body weight and limb lengths, every individual is operating at a different overload. For example, some very obese individuals are unable to chin themselves even once on a horizontal bar. When these individuals attempt this exercise they overload the flexor muscles of the arms to a maximum. Body type plays such a key role in attempts to overload the muscle through calisthenics that very seldom can the overload be increased gradually or systematically. It is difficult, therefore, to improve muscle strength in specific regions of the body.

On the other hand, there are certain advantages to a program of calisthenics which are unique and which make them necessary to any program of strength-building. A general calisthenics program aims to improve metabolism, circulation, relaxation, and general muscular development. It is true that many of these aims can be attained in a sports program. However, a program of sports such as softball, tennis, or baseball, demands more than one person for successful participation, whereas a calisthenics program can be an individual effort and can be followed for a short period of time each day. Such economy of time plus the fact that one can participate with complete independence are very desirable features.

To maintain maximum flexibility in the joints it is important to stretch the muscle groups on each side of the joint. This stretching of the muscles can best be achieved in a program of calisthenics. Touching the toes stretches the hamstring muscle group behind the knees. Knee-bends stretch the quadricep muscle group in the thighs. Many other calisthenic-type exercises are designed for stretching. These exercises increase the temperature and the blood circulation of the muscles and probably decrease the viscosity (resistance to change) of the muscle, thereby preventing injury to the muscle when it is called upon for vigorous contractions. General calisthenics for warm-up and stretching the antagonistic muscles are therefore recommended before any vigorous activity.

ISOMETRICS

A method of strength development which attains an overloading of the muscle by matching one part of the body against another in a virtual tug of war, or push-and-pull contest, is called isometrics. The system has received widespread publicity as a result of E. A. Muller's[1] work in Germany. This is a type of muscular contraction in which the muscle does not decrease in length, as opposed to an isotonic contraction which results in the muscle shortening and the incurrence of movement. According to the reports, a single daily isometric contraction of a muscle continued for six seconds and demanding only two-thirds of its maximum strength will result in maximum strength gains.

Programs of isometric exercises have been devised which exercise each of the major muscle groups of the body. One example is to place the right hand on the side of the head and to push the head sideward, resisting with the right arm.

[1] "The Regulation of Muscular Strength," *Journal of the Association for Physical and Mental Rehabilitation,* 11 (1957), 41.

Hold the tension for six seconds. This exercise develops the muscles of the right side of the neck.

Subsequent experiments have been somewhat inconsistent in supporting all of Muller's theories, and there is still a question as to how many contractions are necessary, and as to the degree of contraction necessary for maximum strength gains.

Until recent years, isometric contractions were used extensively by physical therapists and others concerned primarily with rehabilitation. A complete program of exercises has been developed using this method, and it is possible for a patient to maintain a high degree of general muscle tone and to improve strength in desired muscle groups considerably. Isometric exercises are also extremely valuable for people who are over fifty years of age and to those who have suffered illnesses, particularly heart attacks.

This method of strength development is very difficult for many involved in athletics to accept. Some football coaches have increased the neck strength of their players by using isometric exercises. These are usually performed in pairs, with one player in an all-four position and the other providing the resistance from a standing position, as shown in Drill 8. Many have used a full program which takes only about five minutes before each practice and have allowed this program to replace the more strenuous and time-consuming weight-training programs. Isometric exercise has received wide acclaim as a strength-building method for athletes, but research over the past several years doesn't substantiate the claims; consequently, much skepticism remains.

There are probably some valid reasons for the coaching skeptics. One of them involves muscular endurance. Even though a six-second contraction of a muscle will build strength in the muscle, there seems to be a definite limitation as to the amount of endurance it will engender. In order for endurance to be improved, the number of repetitions would probably have to be increased considerably.

Another question coaches ask is, "Does this type of exercise decrease flexibility?" Because the joint does not move through its full range in the isometric exercises, there seems to be a good possibility that the increase of strength cannot be properly applied to athletics that require free and easy movement. This question needs much study.

Another factor that makes this method of strength development questionable has to do with motivation. How can a coach know if a boy is giving a three-quarter contraction or a full contraction, or is merely going through the motions? In performing the exercises there is no immediate goal, and as a result only the most conscientious players derive the full benefits. There are tests for various muscle groups, such as: (1) a vertical jump for extensor muscles of the leg, (2) a distance throw for arm extensors, and (3) chinning the bar for arm flexors. Other muscle groups may be tested with dynamometers or tensiometers. These tests, however, are quite often too remote from the exercise itself and progress is usually too slow to retain enthusiasm in a large group.

There are many problems to be considered in the isometric exercises, but there are also many possibilities that should be explored by coaches and teachers. The isometric program, coupled with a program of sports, might result in an increase in strength from the first program and an increase in endurance, circulation, and flexibility from the second. To insure further flexibility some stretching exercises can be included in the exercise program.

ISOMETRICS WITH WEIGHTS

Isometrics with weights is the name of a system of exercise which attempts to combine two methods of training, isometrics and isotonics, into one strength-producing system. The exercises are performed with special apparatus known as the Power Rack, illustrated in Figure 2. The illustrated model has adjustable pins, so that the bar can be moved at least a couple of inches up and down. Some models allow more movement. Weights are added to the ends of the bar. Varying amounts of weight can be placed on each end of the bar as desired for an exercise, and the bar can be moved up and down to strategic exercise positions by placing the pins in different holes.

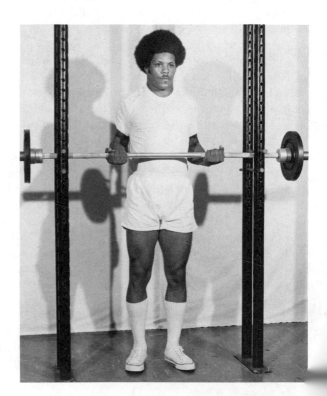

Figure 2. Arm flexion exercise using power rack.

The first phase of an exercise is performed by pushing or pulling the weighted bar against the top pin. The second phase is holding it firm against the top pin (or off the bottom) for a specified time. The bar should be held against the top pin from five to ten seconds. We use seven. If one is working with a heavy overload, a rest period of approximately two minutes is desirable between exercises.

The bar can be set at different pin positions according to the exercise to be performed and the height of the exerciser. Beginners should begin with relatively light weight and should exercise the arms and shoulders first, the back second, and the legs next. As experience is gained during the first couple of weeks, the weight load for each lift should be increased to the maximum that can be held against the top pin for seven seconds. When this can be achieved with a particular exercise, the weight load is increased for that exercise and the sequence altered.

Several precautions should be taken. To avoid back strain one should position himself so that the lifts are performed with the back slightly arched and the hips slightly forward. For best results, it is necessary to exercise specific muscle groups and refrain from "cheating" by bringing into play the larger muscles unless they are being exercised directly. Although some advocates of isometrics with weights maintain that a warm-up is not necessary, the writer recommends a brief program of calisthenics or a light weight program with the power rack, operating with 60 to 70 percent of maximum poundage at each position.

Isometrics with weights is not recommended as a complete weight-training program. It does not have the advantage of exercising through a full range of motion, and thus contraindicates flexibility. It is, however, an excellent supplement to the weight-training program and it is recommended that it be incorporated into the programs in later chapters as an option.

During the off-season when the athlete is concentrating completely on strength and power development, he should work one day with a regular weight-training program and on alternate days practice the skills of the sport in which he is trying to improve his proficiency. If a more concentrated program of strength development is desired, a routine such as that outlined below has been used successfully.

Monday — regular weight-training routine

Tuesday — skill drills for the desired sport followed by isometric routine on the power rack

Wednesday — Same as Monday

Thursday — Same as Tuesday

Friday — Same as Monday and Wednesday except decrease repetitions and increase weight

Saturday — heavy sport skill workout

Sunday — rest

The power rack exercises can be adapted to a variety of training programs as one becomes experienced. A basic program is shown below. Additional exercises and repetitions may be added as the athlete desires and as his needs become apparent. In some cases the program might be too heavy as an alternate routine. In that event it is suggested that only the curl, overhead press, upright rowing, and dead lift be performed.

Exercise	Exercise Angle
1. Curl — elbow-joint angle	$90°$
2. Overhead press — elbow-joint angle	$90°$
3. Upright rowing — elbow-joint angle	$135°$
4. Dead lift — knee-joint angle	$135°$
5. Bench press — elbow-joint angle	$90°$
6. Heel-raise — foot angle	$135°$

Isometric Program with Weights Using the Power Rack

ISOKINETICS

Isokinetic exercise is a method of exercising a muscle so that the resistance to the muscle is determined by the force of the muscular contraction. This is done through an apparatus which adjusts to the force the exerciser applies when either pulling or pushing against the apparatus. The apparatus resists with exactly the same force the exerciser applies, and in so doing, regulates the speed of the contraction. Figure 3 illustrates how the arm flexors can be exercised through a full range of motion using isokinetics.

Phenomenal results have been attained using the isokinetic exercises. The University of Indiana swimming team, 1972 National Collegiate Athletic Association champions, has used isokinetic exercises extensively. Len Dawson, Kansas City Chiefs quarterback and Joe Namath, New York Jets quarterback reportedly have used isokinetics in rehabilitating injured knees.

There are several advantages to isokinetic exercises:

1. Soreness is minimized.
2. The entire program requires very little time.
3. It is virtually injury-free.
4. The apparatus is easily operated.

There are also some disadvantages:

1. The apparatus is fairly expensive.

2. When used by large groups, the apparatus in some instances hasn't held up.

The manufacturers of the apparatus are making constant improvements, however, and basic isokinetic equipment is a recommended addition to any weight room. Isokinetic exercises are highly recommended as a supplement to the weight-training program on a group or individual basis and lend themselves splendidly to rehabilitation exercises.

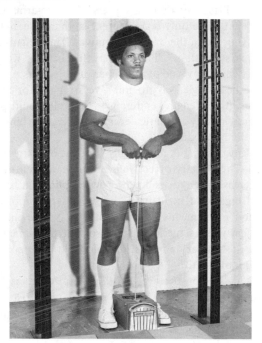

Figure 3. Upright rowing exercise using isokinetic equipment

METAL SPRINGS AND RUBBER CABLES

These two pieces operate on the same principle. The apparatus consists of two handles joined by a series of metal springs or rubber cables. When the handles are pulled apart the springs or cables stretch (expand). The muscle groups can be rapidly overloaded to their maximum by adding to the number of springs or cables. The manufacturers have developed a series of exercises with this apparatus which provide exercise for most of the large muscle groups of the body. The overload can be controlled to a finer degree than with calisthenics, but not nearly so exactly as with weights. This type of apparatus is used chiefly or exercise in the arm and shoulder region because exercises for the leg and ınk muscles are rather awkward.

WEIGHT LIFTING AND WEIGHT TRAINING

There is little distinction to be drawn between weight lifting and weight training. Both involve the lifting of barbells or dumbbells, and when weight is continually added to the bar, both will result in strength gains. The term "weight lifting" has come to mean competitive lifting, whereas "weight training" refers to an interest in physical fitness or improvement in strength for a particular sport. The end result for a weight-lifter is lifting maximum poundage using the three basic lifts: the two-arms press, the two-arms snatch, and the two-arms clean and jerk. The only real differences, therefore, between weight training and weight lifting are in the overall objectives. The weight-lifter lifts weights in order to increase strength so that he may lift heavier weights, whereas the weight trainer may have any one of a number of objectives.

The best single way to improve strength for athletic performance is by lifting weights. Strength, endurance, flexibility, and power are factors of great importance in any athletic event. All can be improved through a sound weight-training program.

Weight training is not usually thought of as an end in itself, but as a means to an end. The primary objective is not to learn to lift as much weight as possible but to increase strength and power for application to some other sport. Unlike weight lifting, form in lifting is of secondary importance except in those lifts where good form means added safety. It is true that each exercise should be done as nearly the same as possible so that the same muscles are exercised each time; but the primary emphasis should be on the power the muscle exerts, not on the form of the lift.

The design of the weight-training program is largely dependent on the sport for which the individual is training. In most sports the emphasis is on explosive power more than strength. Thus most athletes practice lifts that stress development of this explosive power. A combination of speed and strength, power is perhaps the most desirable quality in most forms of athletics. Those individuals using programs emphasizing power usually perform lifts with a lighter weight than weight-lifters and usually perform the exercise with a thrust rather than a deliberate motion. A good example is the substitution by the weight trainee of jump squats for the full squat exercises as shown in Figure 25. Full squats are a more deliberate action than jump squats and much more weight can be lifted. Jump squats are usually performed a greater number of times, with the primary emphasis being placed on the height of the jumps or the thrust of the jumper.

A good weight-training program is a combination weight-lifting and exercise program. The workout should begin with several flexibility-type exercises such as toe touches, squats, arm circling, alternate toe touches, twists, and so forth. These should be followed by a series of lifts with light weights emphasizing those lifts which involve a full body action such as the clean and press, the high pull to chin, the jump squats and the sit ups. The trainee is usually perspiring after this rather demanding warm-up and there is little danger of a muscle pull in the regular lifting program if the lifters don't allow themselves to cool off. The regular lifting program varies from day to day in emphasis and length of workout. In such a program a trainee should improve in speed, strength, power, flexibility, and endurance. Flexibility and power are particularly stressed.

There are some noteworthy advantages in training with weights over the other types of strength training. Because the weights can be added to the bar in small amounts, it is very easy to control the resistance to the working muscles. By recording the amount of weight lifted each day, the trainer is able to gradually and accurately increase the overload of a muscle group during a workout and from one workout to the next. This assures a continuity of strength gains in desired areas. Such gains should be recorded on a chart so that the trainee is able to maintain a running account of his progress.

There are lifting exercises to develop strength for all of the major muscle groups of the body. Using weights, it is easy to concentrate on any muscle group that seems necessary for the training of an exerciser. For instance, the basketball player develops the jumping muscles (leg extensors) with the jumping squats. The football player develops the muscle covering the shoulder (deltoid) with overhead presses. The baseball player develops the wrists with the wrist curl and the reverse wrist curl. In this way strength can be added in specific areas by concentrating some exercises on those muscle groups. It should be noted, however, that it is not considered wise to distort muscle balance. There is a danger of muscle strain, tear, and faulty body alignment if one group of muscles is strengthened out of proportion to the others. Therefore, the best program is one that calls for a workout of *all* the more important muscle groups, with a concentration on the desired areas.

THE EFFECT OF WEIGHT TRAINING ON THE ATHLETE

Weight training done in a haphazard, irregular, and sloppy fashion will not reward a player with satisfactory results. As in most endeavors, he will gain strength and muscle from weights proportionately to the effort he puts forth. If he does not give weight training a sincere effort, there will be little or no gain in strength, and the chances are that he will only realize some sore muscles for his efforts. On the other hand an athlete can derive a great deal of strength, power, endurance, and general fitness by lifting weights in a conscientious manner and on a regular schedule. There is absolutely no better way to improve strength and power for application to all sports and to all walks of life than by training with weights.

Strength

The most obvious and most valuable assets to be derived from lifting weights are gains in strength and power. Experts agree that strength gains are dependent on three factors: (1) the amount of stress applied to the muscle (2) the length of time the stress is applied, and (3) the frequency with which the stress is applied. Very few programs of resistive exercise or of sports are designed to satisfy these criteria so well as weight training. In training with weights the load on the muscles can gradually be increased and a record of progress can be recorded accurately. The number of repetitions or the duration of the overload effort can be controlled and accurately recorded, as well as the frequency of the training sessions. Few modern sports overload the muscles with a heavy resistance. Therefore, very few build strength in muscles even though all demand strength for successful participation.

It is difficult to predict the rate of growth of muscles. We know that strength is roughly proportional to the girth or circumference of muscle, but individuals are so different in initial strength and build, strength-building regimens are so varied, and diets and living habits are so different, that it is impossible to know how rapidly a weight trainer will develop in size or strength. In testing various groups over the past several years it has been found that the increase in strength is quite rapid the first few weeks, after which the gains begin tapering off. As they become stronger the increases in strength become much more difficult. The immediate strength gains are often little more than the result of learning the skills of lifting.

Many efforts have been made to determine the increase in girth measurements a weight trainer might reasonably expect. Again the problem is complicated by differences in types of lifting programs and differences in the amount of muscle and fat in different body types. It is generally believed that when heavy weights are used for an exercise, so that only a few repetitions can be performed, muscle size and strength are increased at the most rapid rate. Some weight trainers encourage lifting weights which can be lifted only three to five times while others believe that the weights should be light enough to be lifted fifteen to twenty times. Those using the heavy weights will usually receive the most rapid increase in girth. We have taken girth measurements of many of our physical education students and athletes over the years. Table 1 shows the changes in girth measurement in one class of 27 Wake Forest University freshmen over a six-week period. These results were obtained with repetitions of eight, nine, and ten. With some groups, we have experienced better results and with others, much worse. However, improvement in girth measuements has been consistent, and one can generally expect to register improvements similar to those indicated in Table 1 if the program is sound and if the effort is honest.

	Number	Before	After	Difference
Age (years)	27	18.26	18.39	
Weight (pounds)	27	148.70	151.30	2.60
Upper arm (inches)	27	11.68	12.47	.79
Chest (inches)	27	36.62	37.55	.93
Abdomen (inches)	27	30.24	30.42	.18
Thigh (inches)	27	19.67	19.97	.30
Calf (inches)	27	13.98	14.10	.12

Table 1. Mean Body Measurements Before and After Six-Week Training Program

Speed

Important to the success of a player in football, basketball, baseball, or track is body speed. Even though speed appears to be an inherent quality, practice will improve technique and coordination so that speed can be significantly improved. Most weight training advocates feel that there are types of weight training exercises which will also improve speed. Many who do not advocate weight training claim that it will impede speed and reaction time. In general, the findings of studies conducted throughout the country have indicated that weight training does not decrease speed; rather, these studies indicate a possible increase. Although there is little information on this question there is an increasing amount of study being done to provide an answer.

In an attempt to add further light on the subject we have begun extensively studying the effect of various types of weight training programs on speed in running. We are experimenting with boys from all skill levels, ranging from groups of the very poorest physical specimens in our freshman physical education classes to our most advanced varsity athletes. No conclusive results have been established, but on the basis of completed tests a speed increase appears to be associated with a concentrated weight training program.

In one experiment a class of 27 of our poorest students was tested on the sixty-yard dash, after which they participated in a supervised weight-training program three days a week for six weeks. During this time they were encouraged to do *no* running. At the end of the six-week period they were retested on the sixty-yard dash. The mean score for the first test was 8.58 seconds, and the mean score for the second was 8.30 seconds, a decrease in time of .28 seconds.

In another experiment the varsity football team did not register the same dramatic results, but did show a marked increase. They were tested on the forty-yard dash in order to approximate desirable football speed. They then participated in a six-week program of weight training, after which they were retested on the dash. The mean score for the first test was 5.68 seconds. The mean score for the second was 5.46 seconds, an improvement of .22 seconds.

Although an adequate solution to this problem is not yet available, there seems to be good reason for believing that weight training can result in greater speed. There is much disagreement as to the type of weight-training routine that will best produce speed, and this difference certainly accounts for some of the variance in findings. Some programs emphasize low repetition, maximum overload lifting, while others adhere to high repetition, low overload lifting. If speed is the desired outcome, speed-type exercisers should be practiced. For this reason a program of rapid lifting with lighter weights apparently offers the best plan for speed development.

Power

Explosive power is the most obvious characteristic of a highly successful athlete. Because power is equal to the product of force times velocity, it is in reality equally dependent on both characteristics of a good athlete, force (or strength) and velocity (or speed). Power can be changed by altering either. A small and relatively weak athlete may, if he possesses great speed, have greater power than a larger athlete who is stronger but slower. He is able to achieve good power by overcoming a shortage of strength with an excess of speed. Conversely, a slow athlete may have great power by overcoming a shortage of speed with superior strength. The most powerful athletes, of course, are those who have exceptional speed and strength. These are the power hitters in baseball, the powerful fullbacks in football, and the rugged backboard men in basketball. They are usually very strong and have the ability to exert explosive bursts of muscular speed.

There are many theories of training to improve power. To be successful all of them must improve either or both of the factors involved; strength and speed. Weight training, sensibly programmed, will develop both factors simultaneously. This is done by overloading the muscle with enough weight to insure strength gains, but not to such an extent that the muscle cannot be contracted successfully with a burst of speed. How this can be done is shown in the following example: In performing the first set of an arm overhead press the lifter presses a weight of approximately 50 percent of his maximum lifting strength ten times, concentrating on speed in thrusting the weight to position. On the second set, weight is added and the repetitions are decreased to eight. On the third set more weight is added and the repetitions are decreased to six. In each set an effort is made to power the weight to a full arm extension position. In this way the muscles are trained for explosive type action. Speed of movement can best be attained by practicing speed with lighter weights, whereas improved strength can best be attained with a maximum overloading of the muscle.

In the study of Wake Forest football players we tested several power items before and after a weight-training program designed primarily to improve power. Leg power was measured using the standing broad jump for distance and arm power was measured using the medicine ball put for distance. In the broad jump the average of the group before the weight-training program was 93.60 inches for 47 players, whereas the average jump after the weight-training program was 94.53 inches, an average gain of almost an inch. In the medicine ball put the initial average was 50.83 feet, whereas the average after the program was 53.76, a gain of almost three feet. These are not astounding gains, but they are significant, and the fact that these highly skilled players improved at all made the program worthwhile. The improvement in lesser-developed individuals would probably be much more dramatic.

Numerous researchers have reported that weight training improves the vertical jump, and some college basketball coaches currently use a variety of weight-training exercises to improve jumping ability. The University of Iowa in the Big Ten Conference was probably the first basketball team to take advantage of this information, and currently many colleges are using weight training to improve leg power.

Numerous baseball players use weight training to improve arm power for hitting and throwing. In another study involving hitting and throwing for distance, we found a significant increase in both skills after a six-week weight-training program. Many other colleges and high schools have resorted to weights to improve arm power for baseball players.

Even though there are men in sports who rank low in strength and power, these men are exceptions and very seldom maintain their positions when faced with competition from more powerful and equally skilled players. Because power can be improved through a good weight-training program, athletes would do well to train to improve power as well as skill. The greatest probable contribution weight training makes to successful participation in football, basketball, swimming, and track and field is increasing power.

Flexibility and Coordination

It has often been said, "Weight training or lifting will result in muscle-boundness or tightening of the muscles." Muscle-boundness is a rather vague term which is also described as a condition that exists because of tense and enlarged muscles and stiff joints. Critics of weight training contend that muscle-boundness is the end result of this type of strength development. They maintain that lifting weights will develop a large, bulky muscle that is slow to stretch, thereby reducing the speed of muscular contraction, flexibility, and coordination.

When light weights are lifted very rapidly a large number of times, the involved muscles are left with a feeling of tightness. This can be overdone to the extent that the muscle becomes congested with blood and feels tight and flushed. Such lifting produces enlarged or "pumped-up" muscles for a short period of time and is accompanied by a decrease in function and strength of the muscle. The tight feeling and extra bulk is soon lost. Advocates of this practice are probably responsible for most of the muscle-boundness stigma attached to weight training for so many years. Intentional "pumping-up" of muscles has no useful place in weight training for sports.

Muscle-boundness is also used to describe the condition of an individual who has concentrated on the development of one group of muscles and completely ignored the antagonistic group. This usually results in an imbalance that seriously impairs any coordinated movement in the area. An example of this practice is the individual who practices only on chins and develops very large and powerful arm flexors. If nothing is done for the arm extensors, the flexors will dominate the extensors so completely that even when the arms hang by the sides they will remain in a partially flexed position. This condition cannot possibly exist if a sensible weight-training program is practiced. Numerous studies are available which generally conclude that weight trainers are *not* less flexible than non-weight trainers, but are more flexible and better coordinated.

Today there is general belief that an individual might become muscle-bound only when he is repeatedly exercising a muscle group in a fixed position. The connective tissues in the muscle become adapted to this position and become shortened.[2] If such a disastrous possibility exists, weight trainers should guard against it by encouraging a full range of motion in the involved joints with each lift. To further develop flexibility, exercises should be used that will require a stretching of the muscles around the joints, because stretching will increase the range of movement of the joint, hence its flexibility. One further precaution to assure that strength and muscle bulk gained from a weight-training program can be applied to a sport lies in encouraging the athlete to practice his sport skills often, especially on the days he is not lifting. If coordination is to be improved for punting a football, then that skill must be practiced. In situations where such a program is followed, the evidence is conclusive that weight trainers are considerably more flexible and better skilled than the average nontrainers.

Psychology

The psychological effect of a player's knowing he is stronger and more powerful than his opponent is a significant feature of his playing ability, whether he is a participant in football, baseball, basketball, golf, tennis, or most any

[2]Laurence E. Morehouse and Philip J. Rasch, *Scientific Basis of Athletic Injuries* Philadelphia: W. B. Saunders Company, (1958). p. 110.

modern sport involving physical activity. Athletes with knowledge of superior physical strength are able to approach a game or match with a feeling of confidence in their physical ability that is immeasurable. Many football coaches brainwash their players into superhuman efforts by selling them on the idea that they are as physically strong as their favored opponents. This strategy often backfires in a game when the realization is hammered home that there is actually a big difference in power. It is much easier to teach mental toughness to an athlete who is already physically tough. Weight training has given some football coaches this added advantage. It has been reported that every starting lineman on the 1958–59 Louisiana State University team could dead lift 400 pounds. If this is true, imagine the psychological advantage those players enjoyed, knowing that they could move a man approximately twice the size of the one they generally faced in Saturday's game. This psychological factor is equally important in other sports. Imagine the feeling of confidence with which muscular Jack Nicklaus enters a golf match, knowing that he can concentrate on accuracy and still outdistance opponents who often press to get equal distance. Ted Williams and Henry Aaron have enjoyed the same type of advantage in baseball. Weight training will assure players added strength and a resulting self-confidence will make an unlimited contribution to successful performance.

Conditioning for Athletics

There is probably no better way for an athletic team to condition or to maintain a high degree of physical fitness than through a sensible weight-training program. In high schools and colleges there are generally restrictions which limit playing seasons in most sports. Because the amount of time in which to prepare for a season is limited, it behooves every coach to encourage his players to report in top physical condition. In this way little actual practice time will be lost because of sore muscles and quick fatigue. Many coaches have found that a satisfactory solution to this problem is a weight-training program approximately six weeks in duration before organized practice sessions begin. Such a program of weight training supplemented with running will pay rich dividends because the boys will have been improving general muscle tone and adding body strength that will prove invaluable after practice begins.

Some sports are of such a nature that a certain movement is seldom used, but when the athlete is called up to perform the movement he has to do so with an all-out effort. For example, a baseball pitcher may go through several games without having to field a slow bunt down the third-base line. When this occasion does arise, the pitcher has to field the ball, stop suddenly, and make a vigorous throw to first. Muscle fibers are called into play that have lain dormant for weeks. Sometimes there is injury to the muscle. To help protect against such injuries, an in-season program of lifting and stretching exercises has been established in some schools. This program is of a modified nature but it helps keep the muscles toned for maximum contractions, and by stretching the antagonist muscles helps maintain a high range of motion in the joints. These exercises will not prevent injury to a muscle that isn't properly warmed up or to one that is being put under sudden stress after it is fatigued. Weight training is only a part of sensible training. It will condition a muscle so that fatigue may be postponed for a far greater length of time. It will also increase the endurance of a muscle many times — but common-sense standards must be observed.

Fitness

If one desires general physical fitness, the easiest and surest way to attain it is with weights. Many claims have been made for weight training, some of which are undoubtedly false. The validity of other claims depends on the type of program and the seriousness of the trainer. However, there are unmistakable benefits to be derived from sensible weight training. These benefits are: (1) improved strength, (2) enlargement of the exercised muscles, (3) improved power, endurance, flexibility, and speed, (4) improved body measurements, and (5) improved confidence and feeling of well-being. The well-trained muscle functions more smoothly and with more power but with less actual effort.

An individual with adequate strength to satisfy his individual needs will use portions of the muscle fibers while the others rest. In this way part of the muscle is able to relax and recover while the other fibers carry the load. Changes in musculature are not automatic. Such things as diet and sleep will greatly influence progress. The trainer must be reasonable enough and serious enough about the entire program to give it a sensible effort. It is not always easy. It's exhilarating to some and work to others, but the benefits mentioned are available to all.

Weight training is of tremendous value to athletes, but the *most* valuable application of weight training is probably in the American home. The stigma attached to weights for so many years has in large part been erased, and there are thousands of sets of weights under beds and in basements throughout the country. Many of these weight owners got started in lifting by training for athletic teams or by lifting in schools and colleges. Because weight training can be so effectively carried into later life it is becoming increasingly important that schools and colleges include it in their regular physical education programs. It is a sport that takes relatively little time or space and requires no additional participants. No other form of physical exercise can approach it for building a fit America.

Controlling Body Weight

Not too many years ago being overweight was looked on as a sign of prosperity. It denoted a comfortable position in life. Today we realize that an obese person may not be well-nourished. We know that excess weight puts an undue strain on our bodies. "Statistics show that people who are very much overweight seem to be more susceptible to certain diseases, may have less resistance to infection, even tend to have more accidents than slim people."[3]

Most diseases of overweight people result from circulatory failures, which now account for a large percentage of all deaths. Weight reduction is a common procedure in treating heart disease, high blood pressure, diabetes, and other life-shortening diseases. Even though overweight is not usually the cause for most of these diseases, weight reduction will often decrease their ill effects.

Weight is primarily bone and flesh, flesh being part fat and part muscle. A person may be overweight because he has large bones, a condition over which one has very little control. Far more often one will be overweight through a surplus of fat or muscle. Such a surplus adds miles of blood vessels to the circulatory system. When one gains weight in the form of fat the burden of supplying this additional weight with blood is almost completely borne by the heart. A gain in weight in the form of muscle is not nearly as burdensome to the heart because the muscles serve as booster pumps for the blood when one is engaged in activity.

Some trainers lift weights in order to gain weight while others lift in order to lose weight. It's confusing that both can be possible. The truth is that neither is possible unless the diet is properly controlled.

Energy is computed in terms of calories which are taken into the body in the form of food. Whether an individual retains or loses weight is dependent on whether the individual converts the energy-yielding calories to energy for exercise or work, or retains it in the form of fat or muscle. Fat is stored energy, a small percentage of which everyone needs, to be used for fuel and heat. If the diet (caloric intake) is held constant and exercise is increased, the calories will be converted to energy and there will probably be a slight weight loss. If the caloric intake is restricted and no exercise is done, weight will be lost according to the degree of limitation on the caloric intake. If the caloric intake is restricted and exercise is increased there will be a weight loss coupled with a toning of the muscles and a redistribution of the weight as fat is converted to fuel. Losing weight is difficult for many people. The caloric intake should be limited through a sensible diet and exercises should consist of light weights with many repetitions. The value of a weight-training regimen in losing weight is its ability to use up calories and to maintain muscle tone and general body fitness.

It is much easier and more natural to gain weight while weight training. In order to gain weight one should eat more (have a higher caloric intake). This is sometimes difficult if one doesn't exercise because the body doesn't need more food. Exercise creates an appetite because it burns a great amount of fuel which must be replaced. Therefore, in order to gain weight one needs plenty of exercise to create a need and desire for food. Exercise will also serve to convert the food

[3]Courtesy of the Metropolitan Life Insurance Company.

to muscle instead of fat. One needs to eat large quantities of the right foods to satisfy the appetite and to get plenty of sleep and rest in order to allow the body time for recovery. Participation in a three-day-a-week weight-training program is an ideal method to exercise when attempting to gain weight.

Strength and Body Weight

There is a relationship between strength and body weight, and if the body weight is largely muscle the degree of relationship is very close. When an individual gains in body weight and gains in strength or lifting power, the added body weight is beneficial muscle. Quite often, however, an individual gains in body weight and does not gain, or even loses, in lifting power. In such cases the increased weight is usually burdensome fat. There seems to be an optimum weight for maximum strength in every individual, a weight anything above which is excess fat and below which is general body weakness. An athlete should be able to maintain an optimum body weight if he diets, competes in his sport, and trains sensibly with weights. Excess weight may not hinder a champion lifter, especially the heavyweights, but it may be troublesome to a football guard who must be fast and agile to be successful. A football tackle may weigh 250 pounds, but there are many men who weigh 250 pounds. To be effective this weight must be muscle capable of explosive power, not fat that hinders movement.

There is an optimal weight for maximum strength in every individual. Many baseball players try to defy this principle by adding weight for greater hitting or throwing power merely through eating more food. If this added weight is considerably above their optimum weight they usually lose more in speed, agility, and endurance than they gain in power. Through weight training and other forms of sports an athlete can control his weight as muscle and concentrate the muscle in areas of the body that need it most.

Strength and Body Build

In most sports the big tall man has a decided advantage. A height advantage plus long arms and legs give him additional range over the smaller athlete, and if height and range are accompanied by strength and speed, his skill is usually beyond the limits of the little man. This is especially true in track, basketball, baseball, and tennis. In lifting weights, however, this type of build puts the athlete at a disadvantage. In lifting he must carry the weight through a much greater arc than the shorter, stockier lifter and also must lift the weight to a greater height. The shorter men have a much better chance to become good competitive lifters even though they may not be nearly so successful in other sports. Also the shorter, smaller men can lift more weight proportionally than larger men. The large man has an advantage in most sports, but in weight lifting the smaller man is most successful.

A knowledge of the relationship of build and lifting strength is valuable to an athlete who is training with weights. Coaches who have their athletic squads training with weights should be aware of these facts so that they might understand why some of their best athletes don't show up well in weight training. The fact that these athletes sometimes cannot excel in lifting weights does not mean that they aren't deriving as much or more benefit from the lifting program. When the strength gained is reapplied to the sport of his choice he will regain the advantage.

The force one is able to deliver is dependent on the length of the limbs, strength, speed, and the angle of pull. Although long levers may prove to be a disadvantage in lifting heavy weights, they are a tremendous asset when the load to be moved is no heavier than a football, basketball, or baseball bat. To use limb length and the angle of pull advantageously the fundamentals of the sport skill must be mastered. Strength and speed are of little advantage when a player is poorly skilled. However, when the player, by practicing his particular sport, learns to use strength and speed he will improve considerably. Strength, speed, power, and form are factors in successful skill performance that cannot be completely separated. Attempts should be made to improve each aspect, not one at the expense of the other. Athletes using weight training should be well aware that improved strength, speed, and power must be applied by using proper technique.

SELECTED REFERENCES

Bunn, John W., *Scientific Principles of Coaching.* Englewood Cliffs, N.J.: Prentice-Hall, Inc., 1955.

Calvin, Sidney, "Effects of Progressive Resistive Exercise on the Motor Coordination of Boys," *Research Quarterly,* XXX (1959), 387-398.

Capen, Edward K., "The Effects of Systematic Weight Training on Power, Strength & Endurance," *Research Quarterly,* XXIII (1952), 361-369.

Chui, Edward, "The Effect of Systematic Weight Training on Athletic Power, Strength & Endurance," *Research Quarterly,* XXI (1950), 188-194.

Councilman, James E., "Isokinetic Exercise . . . A New Concept in Strength Building," *Swimming World,* X, No. 9 (September 1969), 4-5.

Johnson, Warren R., *Science & Medicine of Exercise and Sports.* New York: Harper & Brothers, 1960.

Karpovitch, Peter V., *Physiology of Muscular Activity,* 7th ed. Philadelphia: W. B. Saunders Company, 1971.

Masley, J. W., A. Hairabedian, and D. N. Donaldson, "Weight Training in Relation to Strength, Speed, and Coordination," *Research Quarterly,* XXIV (1953), 308-315.

Massey, Benjamin H., and Norman L. Chaudet, "Effects of Systematic Heavy Resistive Exercise on Range of Joint Movement in Young Males," *Research Quarterly,* XXVII (1956), 41-51.

Massey, Benjamin H., Harold W. Freeman, Frank R. Manson, and Janet A. Wessel, *The Kinesiology of Weight Lifting.* Dubuque: Wm. C. Brown Company, 1959.

McCardle, W. D., and J. R. Magel, "Isometric vs. Isotonic Training," *Scholastic Coach,* XXXIX, No. 2 (January 1970), 32-34.

Morehouse, Laurence E., and Augustus T. Miller, *Physiology of Exercise,* 3rd ed. St. Louis: The C. V. Mosby Company, 1959.

Morehouse, Laurence E., and Philip J. Rasch, *Scientific Basis of Athletic Training.* Philadelphia: W. B. Saunders Company, 1958.

Wilkin, Bruce M., "The Effect of Weight Training on Speed of Movement," *Research Quarterly,* XXIII (1952), 361-369.

4

DEVELOPING
THE WEIGHT-TRAINING
PROGRAM

The number of people participating in a weight-training program may range from one to well over one hundred students and athletes. The amount of equipment purchased should be determined by the following: (1) the expected number of participants in the program, (2) the amount of money available, and (3) the size and arrangement of the facilities. The barbell and two dumbbells are basic equipment. With them a complete training program can be very successfully conducted. On the other hand, the group with a large budget can find an inexhaustible supply of accessory equipment through available magazines and catalogs. Some of this equipment is recommended, but purchase of large amounts is unwarranted since there is little time to use accessory equipment during a supervised program.

EQUIPMENT

Basic Equipment

1. *Barbells.* The barbells should be the first item purchased. They are necessary for any successful program. The barbell is simply a steel bar four to seven feet long with collars that are held to the bar by screws. The collars hold the weights in place at each end and some companies provide a metal sleeve or hand grip that revolves on the bar between the weighted ends. Standard sets usually contain weighted plates of 1¼, 2½, 5, 10, and 25 pounds.

The number of barbells and the amount of weight to purchase depend entirely on the type of program planned. If high school athletes are to be trained and the weights are also to be used in physical education classes we recommend one bar and 150 pounds of weights for every four students. A college group needs 175 pounds of weights for each bar. The five-foot bar with collars weighs 25 pounds, making the total weight available to each group 175 pounds for high school students and 200 pounds for those in college. Some groups will lift more weight in some lifts, and in such instances can borrow weight from other groups. This practice disrupts organization, however, and if possible enough weight should be purchased to discourage it.

2. *Dumbbells.* Most dealers include with a barbell set a pair of 14- to 16-inch solid steel dumbbell bars with revolving hand grips. Outside collars at the ends of each dumbbell hold the weights in place. The same weighted plates are used on the dumbbell bars as are used on the barbell bars.

3. *Bench.* It is a good idea to have a bench of sturdy construction for each group of trainees. It should be twenty inches in height, ten inches wide, and at least six feet in length. The proper size will permit boys of all sizes to perform a bench press without undue restriction in the shoulders and will enable three members of the group to sit and rest as the fourth member is lifting. The height of the bench is the least important factor. Twenty inches is recommended so that the benches may be used to administer the Harvard Fatigue Laboratory Test of Physical Fitness.

Barbells and dumbbells can be purchased in most sporting goods stores or directly from a number of manufacturers. It is best to get competitive bids before buying, especially if one plans to buy in quantity. Consider the freight expenses if buying directly from the factory. If shipped long distances a large quantity of weights can be a major expenditure.

It is possible to have weights made at a foundry or to make them at home from tin cans filled with cement. These are inexpensive ways to get started. However, if you plan to add to the weight room it is best to get the weights from a reputable manufacturer. In this way most of the weights and accessory equipment will be uniform, and as you add to the room a neat appearance will be maintained.

Accessory Equipment

Many equipment devices can be used to advantage when working with a small number of individuals, but only a few are of value with large weight training groups. Some are valuable items used to help build up specific muscle groups for better athletic performance and others are particularly useful for prevention of injuries and rehabilitation after injuries. The school budget will usually permit the purchase of the essential weight-training equipment and such items as the barbells and dumbbells should be bought from a manufacturer. There are, however, many pieces of equipment which can easily and economically be constructed in the school shop or elsewhere.

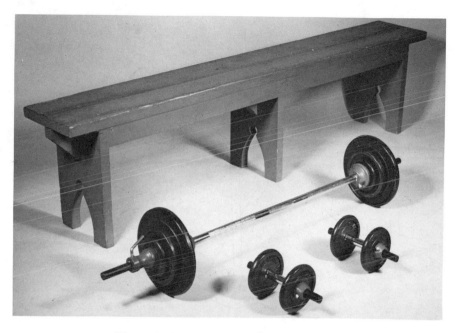

Figure 4. Basic weight-training equipment

1. *Knee Flexor and Extensor Table.* The padded table has an arrangement of bars at one end. Weights are added to the bars in such a manner that the player can sit on the end of the table with his feet under the bar. The knee extensor muscle groups can be exercised by placing the feet under the bar and straightening the leg. The knee flexors can be exercised by lying on the stomach and placing the heels under an additional bar, bending the leg and holding the weights as shown in Figure 5. This table is far more expensive than an iron shoe but it is also much more effective in the treatment of injured knees. It is also available as an isokinetic exerciser. The rope apparatus is attached to the lower bar in place of the weights. There is also a model using a hydraulic cylinder which attaches to the lower bar and regulates resistance.

2. *Bench Press Stand.* Two upright pipes are attached to each side of a heavy bench similar to the rest bench previously described. A Y-shaped cradle should be welded to the top of each pipe to hold the bar while weights are being added. The pipes should extend a comfortable distance above the bench but not so far that boys with short arms can't reach the bar. The bench press exercise develops primarily the arm extensor and chest muscles.

3. *Chinning Bar.* Most gymnasiums are equipped with a standard chinning bar that can be raised or lowered. If the weight room is separate and a chinning bar is not available, it can be easily constructed. A 1½-inch horizontal pipe approximately 3 feet long is attached to the wall with flanges at least 8 feet

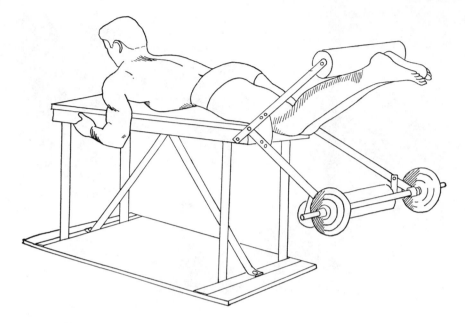

Figure 5. Knee flexor and extensor table

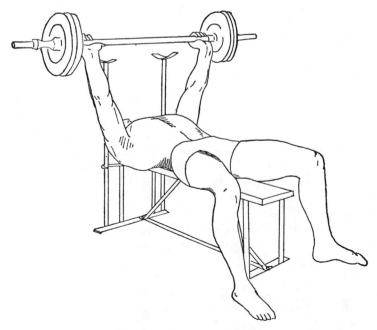

Figure 6. Bench press stand

above the floor. At the opposite end the pipe should attach by means of an elbow to a 1½-inch vertical pipe. The vertical pipe should be secured to the floor or ceiling by a flange. Chinning serves a useful purpose in developing the arm flexors and is a very good self-testing item.

4. *Shoulder Dip Bars.* The construction of these bars is very similar to the chinning bar. Two 1½-inch pipes, 3 feet in length, are attached to the wall 4½ to 5 feet above the floor and 24 to 30 inches apart. They are supported at the wall by flanges and at the opposite end by horizontal 1½-inch pipes. The shoulder dip bars are more economical in space and money than the parallel bars. The shoulder dip exercises develop the extensor muscles of the shoulder and arms.

5. *Knee Bench.* The knee bench as designed by Klein[1] is an excellent knee strengthener. A strong bench 72 inches long and 12 inches wide is needed. An adjustable foot bar is attached in front of the bench so that the player may sit on the bench and place the top of his feet under the foot bar. When he contracts the knee extensors the legs straighten and the body is raised from the bench. The knee bench can be used with very good results to strengthen the extensor muscles of the knee to prevent injury.

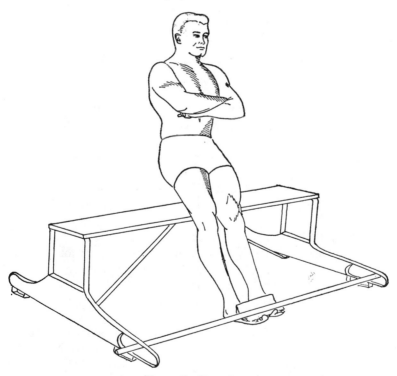

Figure 7. Knee bench

[1]Karl K. Klein, "Specific Progressive Exercise as a Mass Technique for Preventive Conditioning and Reduction of Knee Injury Potential in Athletics," *Journal of the Association for Physical and Mental Rehabilitation.* 10 (1956), 185–189.

6. *Wrist Rollers*. For hand and forearm development the wrist roller is an excellent and inexpensive piece of equipment. A ½-inch hole is drilled through a cylindrical handle 12 inches long and 1½-inches in diameter. A 4-foot rope or window sash cord is inserted into the hole and a knot is tied to secure it properly. A weight is tied to the opposite end. The exercise is performed by rolling the rope onto the handle until the weighted end reaches the handle.

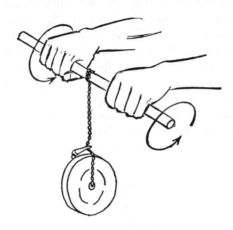

Figure 8. Wrist roller

7. *Scales*. Doctor's scales with an attached height rod are desirable. If the scales do not include a height rod, height can be easily measured by attaching a measuring tape to the wall.

8. *Clock*. A large clock with a minute sweep hand should be attached to the wall in a clearly visible location.

9. *Bulletin Board*. The board should be large enough to post lifting programs for all sports, current events in weight training, progress charts, and so forth.

10. *Multiple-Use Machine*. This fascinating piece of equipment has found its way into weight rooms all over the country. Variations of this machine are available with as many as fifteen stations. The initial cost is high but maintenance is minimal and theft of weight plates isn't a problem. It also has a very good safety record. If space is a problem this machine can accommodate the largest number in the smallest area.

11. *Isometric Power Rack*. This equipment was described on page 20. It is used for functional isometric exercises and is a must for strength development for athletics. If sufficient funds are not available to purchase the racks, they can be constructed by drilling oversized holes in four by fours so that the bar from a barbell set can be used.

Additional Accessory Equipment

Equipment	*Purpose*
1. Anatomical wall charts	Useful for instruction regarding the body musculature.
2. Record forms	Can be printed. A form should be available for each player.
3. Calf machine	Development of the calf muscles.
4. Chalk box	A chalk box with an attached towel should be centrally located to enable the player to dry his hands before lifting.
5. Head strap	Development of the flexor and extensor muscles of the neck.
6. Incline bench	Aid in developing the arm and chest muscles.
7. Iron shoe	Used primarily to strengthen the muscles of the thigh and calf.
8. Knee bend stand	Aid in developing the muscles of the thigh and calf.
9. Latissimus Dorsi machine	Development of the shoulders and upper back. It is especially valuable for swimmers.
10. Leg press machine	Development of the knee and hip extensors.
11. Wall pulleys	Aid in exercising the arms, shoulders, chest and upper back.

FACILITIES

Location

As a rule the weight training room is an abandoned storage room or a corner of the gymnasium floor. Ideally the room for weight training should be separate from the gymnasium floor and located on an outside wall with windows for ventilation and an outside door so that during the warmer months the training groups can be encouraged to work outdoors. The room should be on the ground floor. If it is located over some other room the noise of dropping weights will disturb its occupants.

Construction

The wall construction should be of a strong material such as brick or ement so that various pieces of equipment can be safely anchored. The floor should be concrete, because a concrete floor will suffer little damage when weights are accidentally dropped. If the gymnasium floor is used, wooden platforms are suggested to protect the floor. (Standard gymnasium mats can be used but it is unsafe to lift while standing on the heavy mats.) If the gymnasium mats are used it is suggested that the player stand on the floor between the mats to lift so that proper balance can be maintained. Rubberized mats or rubber foot

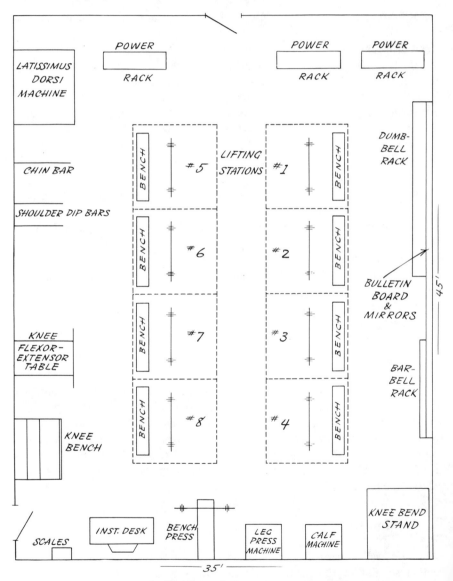

Figure 9. Weight-training room arrangement

matting are very good. The room should be light in color and efficiently ventilated and heated.

Dimensions

The dimensions of the room will vary with the type of program and the number of people that will use the room at one time. If the weight-training room is to be available to athletic teams and physical education classes it should be large enough to accommodate at least thirty-two trainees. Eight groups of four trainees each need an area 7 feet square. This amount of space allows adequate room for a resting bench and a lifting area for each group. The ceiling should be high enough so that the tallest boys may perform the jump squat exercises and the vertical jump tests without touching the ceiling. A room 35 by 45 feet is large enough to adequately take care of thirty-two players, leaving sufficient space around the lifting area for special equipment. Small areas should not be overcrowded with accessory equipment.

Arrangement

There are many ways to arrange the weight-training room. The arrangement shown in Figure 9 is a suggestion based on the actual arrangement of our weight-training room. The room is designed for athletic weight-training groups and for physical education classes. There is no exact pattern for arranging the special equipment along the walls. The scales and the instructor's desk should be conveniently located near the inside door. The arrangement of lifting stations can be varied but care should be taken to place the benches in such a position that the bench press exercise can be performed without congestion. There should be a set of weights at each station. Otherwise the arrangement is a matter of convenience.

If a multiple-use machine is included it should be placed in the central area and should replace at least four lifting stations.

DESIGNING THE PROGRAM

Warm-Up

Before any weight is lifted there should be a vigorous warm-up period of 6 to 8 minutes. The warm-up may be in the form of calisthenics or may be a combination of calisthenics and light lifting exercises. If a calisthenic type warm-up is used it should include some exercises that stimulate general body circulation and others that particularly emphasize stretching exercises of the primary muscle groups. An example of an adequate warm-up period of calisthenics is shown below.

Exercise	Value	Repetitions
1. One-lap jog around track	Stimulate circulation and raise body temperature	1
2. Side-straddle hop	Stimulate arm and body circulation	20
3. Trunk rotation	Increase spine flexibility	10 (right & left)
4. Neck rotation	Increase neck flexibility	10 (right & left)
5. Toe-touch	Stretch low back muscles and muscles behind knees	15
6. Squat thrust	Stimulate leg and trunk circulation	15
7. Arm circling	Increase shoulder flexibility	10 (right & left)

Many coaches have found a combination calisthenics and light weight-lifting program to be the most effective warm-up. The lifts used involve a full body movement and speed and power are emphasized using the light weights. The calisthenics improve flexibility and stimulate circulation. A good way to organize such a program is to retain all of the calisthenics listed in the previous example with the exception of the toe touches. The number of repetitions for each exercise should be cut to one-half the original number and three- or four-power type weight training exercises should be added, such as the following:

Exercise*	Repetitions
1. Modified clean & press	10
2. Squat jump	10
3. High pull-up	10
4. Power curl	10

The barbells should be loaded with the desired amount of weight for each exercise and placed at four stations. The squad should be led through the warm-up routine by the instructor for the first few sessions but they should be encouraged to go through this part of the program independently as soon as it seems feasible. The exercises should be taken in the order listed so that congestion at the barbells can be partially eliminated. Discourage straggling, or those who finish first will cool off before the actual lifting program begins.

*See Chapter 5 for a description of the exercises.

Determining Starting Weights

There are several good methods for determining the weight with which a player should start, all of which are trial and error to some degree. The easiest, though not the most accurate, method is one based on weight and body build. These factors can serve as a very rough estimate of strength and can be used to facilitate getting boys started. The following starting weights are proposed on the assumption that the trainee is healthy, reasonably strong for his age and size, and has never done any previous weight training:

Exercise*	Suggested Starting Weight
1. Clean and press	One-third of body weight plus ten pounds
2. Sit-ups	No weight
3. Bench press	One-half of body weight
4. Half-squat or leg press	One-half of body weight plus ten pounds
5. Curls	One-third of body weight plus ten pounds

When body weight is the criterion used to establish initial loads, the overweight boy will often find the suggested loads too heavy. A more accurate way to get the program started is to subjectively divide the squad into groups of four for each listing station. This can be done according to height or weight, grouping boys of the same size. Have them sit at the lifting stations while they are shown how to count the weight and properly change the weights on the bar. Then have each group take all the weight off the bar at their station and await further instructions.

Demonstrate the overhead press. Have each player perform this exercise properly with the empty bar to get the feel of the lift. Two members of the group hand the bar to a third at a chest-high position while the fourth member sits at the rest bench. After one member performs the lift they rotate until every member of the group has lifted. Each one lifts, assists and rests with each weight change. Then proceed, in 20-pound jumps, to add weight until the players appear to be nearing their limit. Drop the increases to 10 pounds and then to 5 until each player fails to complete the lift. When a player has lifted his maximum he remembers that figure and continues to help until all members of his group have completed the test. At that point, the coach calls the roll and records each player's best lift. All lifts should be done correctly, with no cheating, if an accurate picture of the lifter's strength is to be recorded. Other lifts usually tested are the three-quarter squat, two-arm curl, and the bench press. Soreness can be minimized if a series of light exercises is performed at the completion of the maximum lifts.

*See Chapter 5 for a description of the exercises.

Another method of getting maximum lifts is to load the bars in 10-pound intervals at different lifting stations around the room. After proper warm-ups and demonstration, have each player start in single file at the lightest weight and execute the desired lift. On completion of the lift he proceeds to the next highest weight and completes the lift, and on up the weight scale until he can no longer perform a correct lift. He is asked to remember his best lift. When everyone has gone as far through the weight scale as possible the roll is called and the players answer with their best lifts. It is not a good idea for an individual working alone to attempt these tests. With no experience in lifting one can easily find himself stuck with a weight and not know how to safely rid himself of it.

Each player's program must be worked out separately on the basis of his maximum lift test. It is best to work out a high-repetition light weight program for the first few sessions. One of the best ways to arrive at a proper beginning weight is to take 40 percent of the player's maximum lift and have him perform one set of ten repetitions. Add 10 pounds and perform another set of ten repetitions.

For example, if a player's maximum overhead press is 100 pounds, his first set of ten is 40 pounds (.40 X 100). His second set is 50 pounds. As the amount of weight increases, the number of repetitions decreases.

The entire program can be calculated for each player on the basis of the four basic lifts. An example of arranging a beginner's program is shown below:

Name: John Doe	Maximum Lift	Starting Weights (Two sets of ten repetitions)
Overhead press	80 .40 X 80 = 32	30-40
Three-quarter squat	120 .40 X 120 = 48	50-60
Two-arm curl	60 .40 X 60 = 24	25-35
Bench press	100 .40 X 100 = 40	40-50

Other lifts compare closely to the ones tested and starting weights for the more popular lifts should be the same as one of those tested. The player will be able to go much faster in some of the lifts but it is a much better practice to start too low than too high. The lifts may be grouped as follows for beginning weights.

1. Overhead press, clean and press, upright rowing
2. Three-quarter squat, dead lift, rise on toes
3. Two-arm curl, stiff-legged dead lift, bent-over rowing
4. Bench press

This method of determining starting weights involves some outside work for the coach or instructor, but it enables him to start the program of lifting o an organized basis the second day of class. Time is a precious commodity with organized weight training, so it is important that only a minimum amount be used for organization and experimentation during actual lifting time.

After the starting weights are determined for each player they should be recorded on a record form such as the one shown in Figure 10. One of the advantages of a weight training program is the ease with which gains in strength can be recorded. If interest is to be maintained it is very important to keep each player's record up to date and to make sure that it is available for his examination.

Selection and Arrangement of Exercises

Exercises should be selected according to the objectives of the specific lifting program. For example, a breast stroker on the swimming team will probably concentrate on the muscles that pull the arm to the body, whereas a baseball pitcher will develop those muscles that thrust the arm away from the body. It is desirable of course to develop the general musculature first and to concentrate on specific muscle groups later. Exercises for the general musculature should include a lift for each major muscle group of the body. There are over 700 exercises that can be done with weights. Quite obviously there is time to perform only a few. These few must be picked carefully. The seven exercises listed below and described in Chapter 5 are considered basic and will satisfy the needs of most beginners:

1. Squats	Upper legs and hips
2. Bench press	Chest and upper arms
3. Stiff-legged dead lift	Back and posterior of legs
4. Heel-raises	Lower legs and ankles
5. Overhead press	Shoulders and posterior of upper arms
6. Sit-ups	Abdomen
7. Two-arm curl	Anterior of upper arms

The above program exercises the major muscle groups of the body and the lifts are so arranged that no two lifts exercise the same muscle groups in succession. This assures adequate recovery time from each lift.

Some exercises can be added and some can be substituted for those exercises on the list as desired. The important point to remember is to start with a basic group of exercises for general body development before concentrating too heavily on individual muscle groups.

Name _____

Training Items		Date		Date		Date		Date		Date		Date	
1. WEIGHT													
2. SQUATS	L.												
	R.												
	L.												
	R.												
3. BENCH PRESS	L.												
	R.												
	L.												
	R.												
4. STIFF-LEGGED DEAD LIFT	L.												
	R.												
	L.												
	R.												
5. HEEL RAISE	L.												
	R.												
	L.												
	R.												
6. OVERHEAD PRESS	L.												
	R.												
	L.												
	R.												
7. SIT-UPS	L.												
	R.												
	L.												
	R.												
8. TWO ARM CURL	L.												
	R.												
	L.												
	R.												

The symbol "L." means weight load; "R." means repetitions.

Figure 10. Weight-training program chart

Grouping

On the basis of the maximum-lift tests the squad should be placed as nearly as possible into homogeneous groups. The strongest should be put in group one at lifting station one; the next strongest in group two at lifting station two; etc. It should be made obvious that the squads have been separated according to strength. This knowledge will serve as an incentive for progressing rapidly in order to move into a stronger group. Remember, these are ability groups and ability should change. To maintain good organization move the players around so as to keep the lifting groups alike. These changes should be made between training sessions and posted so that there will be a minimum of confusion. Do not permit the boys to wander from one group to another during training sessions. This practice disrupts the general organization.

After the squad has been grouped according to strength, an exercise chart should be assigned to each group. These should list each group member's weight, a list of exercises to be performed, the amount of weight to be lifted, the number of sets, and the number of repetitions in each set. It is best to have these charts available at all times during the training session so that the boys can study them during their rest periods. It is very important that the chart be kept up to date. This can best be done by having the players inform the coach when they are ready to move up. The coach then makes the change in the schedule, giving him an opportunity to check the progress of each player and offer advice or encouragement.

Within the groups some further organization is necessary. The group member using the least amount of weight will start the exercise. Two boys will assume positions at each end of the bar to act as loaders. The fourth member sits on the bench. The lifter calls his weight to the loaders as his turn to lift comes up. When the bar is properly loaded and the lift is completed the lifter takes his place on the bench for a brief recovery period. The boy on the bench will replace one of the loaders, who moves to the other end of the bar. The other loader takes his place at the bar to begin lifting. The group will continue to rotate in this fashion until the exercise is completed. Each boy should check the exercise chart while on the rest bench to determine the amount of weight he will use for the next lift. The following exercise is started and conducted in the same manner. The loaders should remain alert to help the lifter if he has difficulty.

Time Allotment

Maximum strength and power gains are realized if the player works hard at lifting for a relatively short period of time. This should be the foundation on which any weight-training program is organized. The time allotted to weight training is usually relatively short so it is very important that players participate in a vigorous routine. The shorter the exercise period the more important it becomes to be so organized that all lifting time can be used to full advantage. An adequate program can be conducted in approximately thirty minutes, but an ideal program will take an hour to an hour and fifteen minutes.

In order to organize properly the instructor must decide on the percentage of the maximum load to be lifted, the number of repetitions to be lifted in each set, the number of sets to be performed, and the amount of time that is needed between sets to recover.

There are two schools of thought regarding the scope of the exercise program for beginners. One recommends that a wide variety of lifts should be included and that only one set of each be performed. This type of program has much merit if time is not a limiting factor. The other group recommends only a few basic exercises to be performed, completing three sets of each exercise. Such a core program of basic exercises enables the player to concentrate on the lifts that exercise the major muscle groups and requires less involved weight-changing on the bar. A combination of the two programs appears to offer the best plan.

Use two sets of ten repetitions for the seven basic exercises during the first two weeks. On the first workout of the third week, the trainee should be ready to add weight, so a new program is appropriate. Add enough weight so that only ten repetitions can be performed with the first set of each exercise (except sit-ups). After completing the first set, weight should be added and the maximum number should be lifted on the second set of all exercises except the stiff-legged dead lift and sit-ups. The last lift of the second set of each exercise should overload the muscles to a maximum. In fact, when the exercise can no longer be performed, the bar should be held isometrically at the all-out position before quitting. After experimenting with many types of programs over the years, it is our feeling that the best results are achieved when there is a maximum overload of the muscles at least every other day.

On the second day (Wednesday) of the third week the same workout should be performed. On the third day (Friday), if time permits, an extra set should be performed in each exercise so that the program would be a set program of 10-maximum-maximum instead of 10-maximum as on the first two days. The bar should be weighted so that the ten repetitions cannot be surpassed in the first two sets. On the third set the last lift should be an all-out effort.

It is not suggested that maximum sit-ups and stiff-legged dead lifts be performed in the early training period. Increase the sit-ups gradually each workout until at least a hundred can be done. The stiff-legged dead lift is an excellent exercise for the lower back muscles, but maximum lifting is not indicated because of the danger of injury. The trainee will have to work up more gradually with this lift and should forego the exercise if low back pain develops.

On the first two days the entire program should be completed in forty-five minutes. The three-set program on Friday can be completed in approximately one hour.

If a muscle group is intensely exerted for a short period of time, that muscle group needs recovery time before it is exerted again, both during the exercise period and between exercise periods. If each exercise is demanding, a rest period of two-and-a-half to three minutes between each set of repetitions is needed.

However, if a beginner starts with 40 percent of his maximum lift and performs two sets of ten repetitions of each exercise, a recovery period of three minutes is not needed between sets. When working in groups of four trainees, the period of time that one waits while three other group members lift is an ideal recovery period. The training program should be so organized that successive exercises involve entirely different groups of muscles, so that the program can continue with no delay.

In order to allow adequate recovery time between lifting sessions, it is recommended that lifting be done every other day. This frequency of lifting is conducive to maximum strength and weight gains and is convenient for an alternate day program of agility and skill drills for athletic squads as well as for a power rack isometric program.

Progression

For the first few days a beginner lifts it is best for him to remain on the two-set program of ten repetitions for each exercise. This gives the muscles an opportunity to become accustomed to strenuous exercise and it gives the player a chance to learn the lifts properly with relatively light weight. After the initial soreness is gone he will add weight when ten repetitions can be performed with the second set. When this can be accomplished, both sets are increased by ten pounds. For example, suppose the player is on a 10-maximum program of 60 and 70 pounds. When he becomes able to lift 70 pounds ten times he is allowed to change his weights to 70 and 80 pounds. When the 80 pounds can be lifted ten times his weights will be changed to 80 and 90 pounds.

After three or four weeks of lifting, it is a good idea to occasionally lower the number of repetitions in each set so that heavier weights can be handled. This can best be done on the last lifting day of the week (Friday if the weight-training days are on Monday, Wednesday, and Friday). On Friday then, the three sets consist of five, three, and one repetitions. The first set of five is the same weight as the second set on the regular lifting days. Ten pounds are added to each set and each player continues to add weight and do one repetition as long as he can do it honestly. Such a schedule is a good routine-breaker and provides the occasional testing the muscles need for maximum strength gains and motivation.

The muscles of the back and legs are stronger than those of the arms and shoulders and are capable of lifting more weight. Weight increases should occasionally be 20 pounds instead of 10 for the lifts involving the larger muscle groups.

Rapid improvement can be expected the first few weeks. This is partly because the players are usually started on a program of conservative weights and will be eager to reach what they consider their actual lifting level. The rapid improvement is also due to improvement in lifting technique and, naturally, an increase in strength. The gradient will gradually level off until near maximal lifting strength is gained.

Eventually the player will reach a "sticking point," or strength plateau, beyond which it seems impossible to go. When this happens a new routine should be tried, and it is sometimes a good idea to stop weight training for a week or ten days. One way of getting past a sticking point is by varying the Friday program as suggested previously. A five, three, one program with heavier weights than normal is very good. Another method is to select a poundage below that at which the player is stuck and repeat three sets of ten repetitions for several sessions.

Alternate-day program

The success of any weight-training program is largely dependent on the amount and type of activity in which the players participate on the days they do not lift. The alternate-day program should fit the individual needs of each player, and for this reason stereotyping is an impossibility. For one who is underweight, it is very important that little physical activity be undertaken on the days he doesn't lift. To gain weight the off day is needed for recuperation and the building of the musculature. For a person of normal weight, or overweight, an alternate-day program should not be deleterious. Everyone should have at least one day during the week in which there is very little physical activity.

For athletic squads training with weights, it is very important that an alternate-day program be followed. Strength and power acquired through weight training can best be applied to a skill if that specific skill is practiced. A basketball player should shoot baskets, dribble, jump, etc., on his alternate day. A football player should kick, pass, pull out, charge, etc., on his off day. If rules prohibit this form of off-season training even on an individual basis, the player should participate in a program of agility and running drills. Handball is an excellent off-day game. Alternate-day programs for various sports are discussed under their respective chapters.

Significant strength gains have been achieved in recent years through the use of the power rack on alternate days. The program should be performed on Tuesdays and Thursdays (assuming that the suggested weight-training routine is followed on Monday, Wednesday, and Friday) after skill and agility drills have been completed. The following basic isometric exercises with weights should be performed holding each for seven seconds; curl, press, upright rowing, bench press, heel-raise, and dead lift. In order to achieve maximum power results, the bar should be loaded close to maximum and should be driven forcefully against the top pin or notch. Because it is performed after the skill program, only minimum warm-ups are usually necessary.

The extent to which the players participate in an alternate-day program depends largely on their physical condition. The underweight athlete should be given a very light workout on the alternate day, but he should not be excused from such a program. The athlete of normal weight should be given a vigorous program lasting from a half-hour to forty-five minutes, and the overweight athlete should be given an even heavier program. Agility and speed-type drills on alternate days are a necessity for the overweight.

Supervision

Some coaches claim that their squads are participating in a weight-training program when in reality there is no program at all. Often the so-called program is handled much as some coaches handle physical education classes: throwing out a ball and letting them play. Enough money is appropriated to buy a couple of sets of weights and they are located in a corner of the gym. A suggested program of weight training is cut from a magazine article and posted on the wall. The squad is called together and lectured on the value of weights. After a demonstration or two they are started on weights. Occasionally the players are asked how they're getting along and, if not doing very well, told, "You'd better get on those weights, you'll need that strength."

If one is tempted to conduct a program of this type, said coach or teacher will be much better off leaving weight training alone. Weight training is hard work. It requires much time and effort to be properly organized, and it thrives best when properly supervised. The benefits of weight training must be interpreted to the players. Techniques must be explained and demonstrated. Routines must be arranged and lifting records must be kept up to date. The players ought to be motivated through contests, variations in the programs, and charts. Publicity should be given the program in local papers. These and countless other jobs are a coach's duty if a successful program is to be conducted. He should decide beforehand if the values that can be derived from weight training are worth such an effort.

The most successful weight-training program is one in which the instructor or coach is present and pushes the boys at a fast pace. Each group should change from one exercise to another at the same time. The instructor should have the exercises written out for each group before the session starts, and during the session he should circulate around the room, offering advice and encouragement, and recording progressions on the exercise charts. Enthusiasm is contagious. A coach's enthusiasm is evident only if he is present and is supervising. If he has some qualified and interested person to supervise the routine the coach should stay in close contact and actively show his endorsement. Regular attendance on the part of each player and the supervisor is necessary for a successful program.

GENERAL SAFETY PRACTICES

Weight training is one of the safest sports. It is only dangerous when carelessness and ignorance replace good judgment and common sense. Grouping by ability, securely fastened weights, proper progression, and various other items previously discussed were closely related to safety. The following comments are directed toward safety and the instructor's responsibility for the standards under which the program will operate.

Medical Examination

The first and most important consideration is the requirement of a complete medical examination prior to participation in a weight-training program. This precaution is no more necessary for weight training than for any other form of strenuous physical exertion, but it should be done before undertaking any athletic or physical education activity. The results of such a physical examination can give assurance that the individual is organically sound. If not, he should be excluded from the program.

When a player returns after injury or illness he should have the same careful examination to determine his capabilities. The player returning after illness or accident will have to be watched to avoid his overdoing the activity in a weakened condition. Conversely, some players may have to be encouraged to exercise an injured limb in order to maintain its strength. Time should be allowed for rehabilitation before resuming heavy work by the injured part.

Lifting Precautions

Correct lifting position is a point the coach or instructor should emphasize repeatedly. When lifting the weight from the floor the correct position is with the feet close to the bar and on the same line, hips lowered, knees flexed, head up, and back straight. The weight should be lifted with the legs, not the back muscles.

Master each lift with lighter weights before attempting to progress to a maximum lift. The time taken to master a lift not only assures proper technique but it also conditions the muscles to lifting, thereby reducing the danger of a pulled muscle. Careless stance, incorrect form, and over-optimism in an effort to show off will result in needless accidents and injuries.

It is important to maintain good discipline in a weight room. Wandering from station to station and engaging in general "horseplay" may result in bumping into another lifter and could result in a serious accident. Everyone should remain clear of those players actually engaged in performing a lift.

Always make certain that the collars that hold the weights in position are securely tightened. Some coaches prefer to use spotters at each end of the bar and dispense with placing the collars in position after each change in weights. Such a system makes it extremely important for the spotters to be in position at the ends of the bar to prevent the bar from tilting.

Many weight-training rooms have weights that are spot-welded to the bar for permanent security and safety. A large number of combinations of weights is necessary for such a program but it eliminates a major safety hazard in weight training.

If straps are used to attach weight, it is advisable to pad such straps with either foam rubber or a felt pad. The weight should be firmly attached to the exercising part and the player placed in the optimal position for performing the exercise.

This precaution is especially important when doing rehabilitative exercises. For example, in performing an exercise with the iron boot it is a must to have the boot firmly strapped, and particular care must be taken not to twist, stretch, or overextend the knee joint. Safety, comfort, and control are essential at all times. If the performer cannot control an attached weight an assistant should be ready to help as needed.

Maintaining Body Temperature

Mention has been made of the need for an adequate warm-up before serious lifting. It should be mentioned that there is also a danger in cooling off too rapidly. Train in comfortable, well-fitting gymnasium clothing, and use appropriate body covering, such as a sweat suit to prevent chilling when the workout is finished. Good organization and supervision keep a program moving at a pace fast enough to prevent cooling off between lifts.

Influence of Gravity

Muscles taxed to capacity and beyond will demonstrate maximal strength gains according to the overload principle. A note of caution is in order for work with such capacity loads. Be careful when swinging loads forward with a ballistic movement and avoid dropping a load under the influence of gravity. For maximum benefit the muscles should be forced to carry the weight smoothly through the full range of the exercise and return it smoothly to the starting point. Concentrate on each exercise and strive for correct performance.

Lifting During Playing Season

Many coaches do not advocate lifting during a sports season. Others follow a modified training program during the season in order to help retain existing strength. Increased strength alone can improve performance, but the coach should use judgment in selecting amounts and kinds of exercise. It is probably unwise to try an increase in lifting ability during the season. Work on a maintenance program which is similar to the regular workouts but do not attempt adding weight to the bar. In-season training programs for specific sports are discussed in later chapters.

Breath Control

No section on safety and supervision would be complete without a comment on breath control while exercising with weights. It is usually advisable to have the performer inhale while engaged in the execution of a particular movement. Forced inhalation aids in fixing the chest walls to provide needed support for the movement of arms and shoulder girdle. He should exhale as he returns to the original position; he must not hold the breath while completing a number of repetitions.

Weights and the Heart

Weight training with heavy loads should not be performed by persons afflicted with cardiac difficulties. The medical check-up prior to participation should catch those with a history of cardiac disturbances and should save the boy and his supervisor from possible danger and embarrassment because of ignorance of a potentially dangerous heart condition. An isometric exercise program is indicated for those individuals. This program, however, should necessarily come from the physician.

Hernia

Interabdominal pressure is also raised during an all-out effort, and for that reason, persons with hernia or a weak abdominal wall should not attempt heavy lifting exercises. An unsuspected hernia may become evident during exercise when a boy complains of a burning sensation or other pain or discomfort in his groin. The supervisor of a weight-training program should be alert to this danger and caution the participants in advance, so they they may inform him if any suspicious circumstances occur.

Trauma

There is seldom any danger of trauma or injury to the muscle fiber as a result of lifting. Physiological deterrents intervene to protect the organic systems of the human body. The psychological limit is usually reached, and the human will fails long before the physiological limit is reached.

Some evidence of trauma to supporting structures such as ligaments and tendons has been found, even though tension usually develops too slowly to produce muscle tears from weight lifting. Ligament and joint injury is more often caused by an improperly performed exercise or by the use of straps to fix loads to the body. Such injuries are usually minor and recovery is spontaneous.

Individual Differences

A word of caution is in order about pushing high school or younger boys too hard. The leader should know the boys and know whom to encourage and whom to moderate. The overweight boy may need encouraging, for according to his size he should, perhaps, be lifting with the stronger when in reality he is lifting with the weaker boys. They, in particular, will need to be assigned extra curls because many of them will be unable to chin themselves even once.

The programs recommended in the following chapters are applicable equally to high school, college, or professional athletes. We have used the same programs with all three groups and there is no good reason to alter those that are offered in each sport solely because of the age differences.

SELECTED REFERENCES

DeLorme, Thomas L., and Arthur L. Watkins, *Progressive Resistive Exercise*. New York: Appleton-Century-Crofts, Inc., 1951.

Massey, Benjamin H., Harold W. Freeman, Frank R. Manson, and Janet A. Wessel, *The Kinesiology of Weight Lifting*. Dubuque: Wm. C. Brown Company, 1968.

Morehouse, Laurence E., and Philip J. Rasch, *Scientific Basis of Athletic Training*. Philadelphia: W. B. Saunders Company, 1958.

Murray, Alistair, *Modern Weight Training*. New York: A. S. Barnes and Company, 1971.

Murray, Jim, *Weight Lifting and Progressive Resistance Exercise*. New York: A. S. Barnes and Company, 1954.

Murray, Jim, and Peter V. Karpovitch, *Weight Training in Athletics.* Englewood Cliffs, N.J.: Prentice-Hall, Inc., 1956.

O'Shea, John P., *Scientific Principles and Methods of Strength Fitness.* Corvallis, Oregon: Oregon State University Book Stores, Inc., 1966.

Paschall, Harry B., *The Bosco System of Progressive Physical Training.* Columbus: Published by the author, 1954.

Randall, Bruce, *The Barbell Way to Physical Fitness.* Garden City, N.Y.: Doubleday and Company, Inc., 1971.

5

WEIGHT-TRAINING
TERMS AND EXERCISES

There are many exercises that can be performed, with or without weights, with hundreds of variations for each exercise. It would be both impractical and impossible to discuss more than a basic list in this chapter. In selecting the exercises for this book three questions were asked: (1) Does the exercise properly overload the muscles with which we are concerned? (2) Is the exercise easy to explain and simple and safe to execute? (3) Does the exercise involve special equipment or involved changes in the barbell or dumbbells? In conducting weight-training workouts with large groups it is very important that they be simple, safe, and quick to administer. More complicated and specialized work should be done in small groups or on an individual basis.

DESCRIPTION OF BODY MOVEMENTS

It is not necessary to be an expert to participate in weight training. However, if one is going to instruct a squad it is very important that he understand the musculature and the joint action of the body in order to design a simple training routine. The nomenclature of joint actions is admittedly confusing because of its inconsistent terminology, but most of the movements have rather familiar terms which can be adequately described.

For the purpose of defining joint actions, it should be assumed that the body is in an anatomical position, which is the erect standing position with the arms hanging by the sides and the palms of the hands facing forward. The fundamental body movements either start from or return to this position.

Flexion and Extension

Flexion is that movement around a joint which decreases the angle formed by the bones at the joint. Extension is increasing the angle of the joint. Flexion and extension are often compared to the hinge on a door. Flexion is closing the hinge, extension is opening it. Trunk flexion is bending over, as in the toe-touching exercise, whereas trunk extension is returning to the original position. If the movement is continued to an arched back position the proper term is hyperextension. Lateral flexion of the trunk is bending the body to either side at the waist.

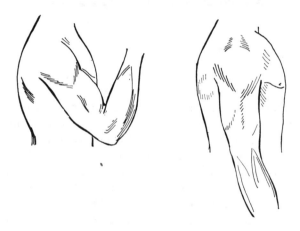

Figure 11. Flexion and Extension of the Elbow

Flexion at the ankle joint means the top or dorsal surface of the foot is lifted toward the front part of the shin and extension means the opposite motion. Flexion of the ankle is also referred to as "dorsi-flexion" and extension is usually called "plantar-flexion."

Abduction and Adduction

Abduction means moving a part laterally away from the midline of the body; adduction is the opposite — moving from a position of abduction back toward the anatomical position. Primary joints for consideration are those of the shoulder and the hip. There is no abduction or adduction in the elbow or knee joints.

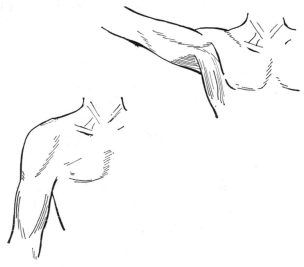

Figure 12. Adduction and Abduction of the Shoulder

Rotation

Rotation is a movement of a part around the long axis of a bone. Inward or medial rotation is the anterior or front surface turning inward; outward or lateral rotation is the opposite. Twisting the head or trunk is referred to as right and left rotation.

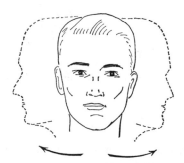

Figure 13. Rotation of the Head

Circumduction

A sequence of movements in which the part describes a cone is circumduction. The apex of the cone is the joint and the open end of the cone is the distal end of the moving bone. Circumduction is a combination movement of abduction, extension, adduction, and flexion, such as the action at the shoulder joint in performing the arm circling exercises.

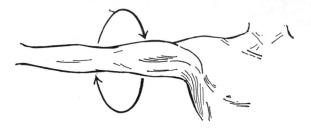

Figure 14. Circumduction of the Shoulder

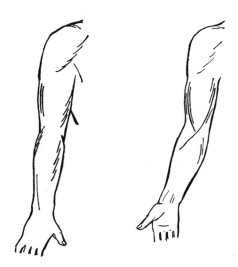

Figure 15. Pronation and Supination of the Forearm

Pronation and Supination

Pronation and supination are movements of the forearm and foot. When the wrist or hand is rotated inward the motion is called pronation; the opposite movement is supination. Pronation of the foot is lifting the outside border or everting the foot; supination is the opposite and is also referred to as inversion of the foot.

Elevation and Depression

These terms are usually interpreted to mean a lifting and dropping of the shoulders. Elevation is lifting the shoulders as is practiced in the shoulder shrug exercise; depression is allowing them to return to normal.

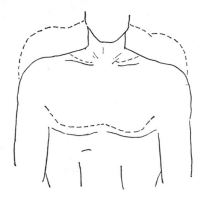

Figure 16. Elevation and Depression of the Shoulders

DESCRIPTION OF LIFTING POSITIONS

The terminology for various weight training movements and lifting positions has common usage, and though slang terms are often used to describe different movements, there is a standard set of terms. No attempt has been made to describe all lifting positions or movements because there are literally hundreds of combinations of positions and movements.

Lifting Grips

1. Overhand – The hands grip the bar so that the palms face toward the legs with the thumbs toward each other.
2. Underhand – This is the opposite of the overhand grip in that the palms face away from the legs as the bar is gripped, and the little fingers are toward each other.
3. Alternate – In the alternate grip one hand takes an overhand grip, the other an underhand grip.

Figure 17. Lifting Grips. (a) Overhand, (b) Underhand, (c) Alternate

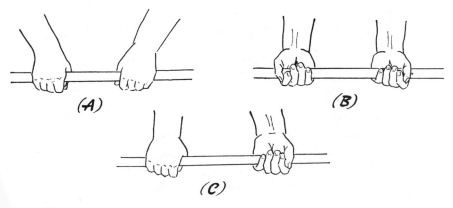

Lifting Positions

1. Standing — For a physical activity in which a powerful force with the upper body is to be delivered, a firm foundation is of great importance. Hitting a baseball, driving a golf ball, or delivering a shoulder block requires stances or positions of the legs and feet that will assure a good base. The basic position for most weight-training exercises has the feet spread about shoulder-width apart and comfortably positioned, either straight ahead or toed-out slightly. The body is erect with arms at the side.

Figure 18. Basic Position

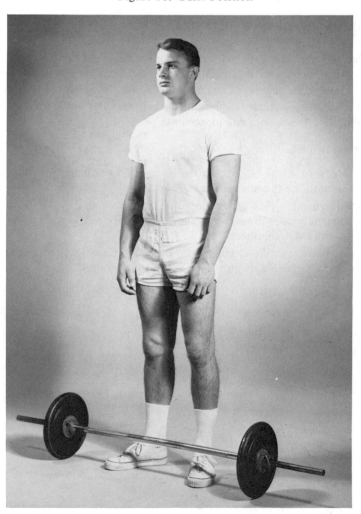

2. Crouch — This position is assumed for virtually all exercises in which the bar is lifted from the floor. Take the standing position with the feet under the bar. Bend at the knees and hips to a crouch position and grip the bar naturally. A check of the crouch position is as follows: arms extended down; hands grasping the barbell outside the knees; head up; knees and hips flexed so that the hips are low; back flat; feet shoulder-width apart, flat on the floor, and comfortably positioned.

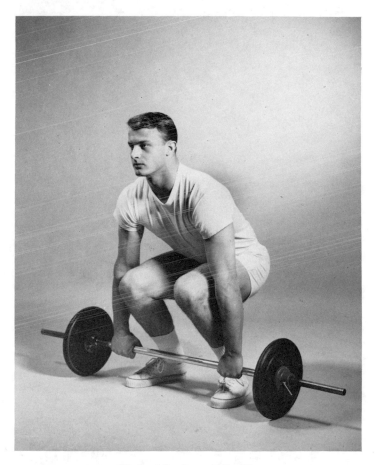

Figure 19. Crouch Position

3. Thigh Rest — The thigh-rest position is the standing position with the chest out and the shoulders back, the arms extended downward allowing the bar to rest against the thighs. The overhand, underhand, or alternate grip may be used.

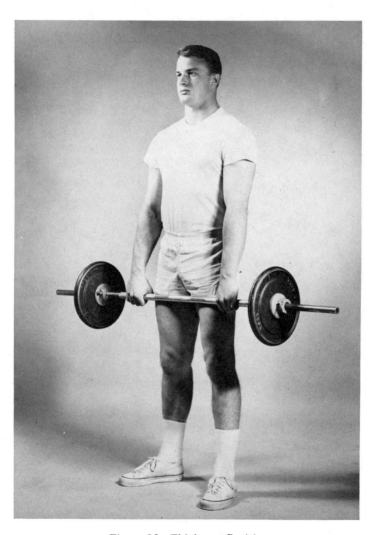

Figure 20. Thigh-rest Position

4. Chest Rest — The bar rests on the chest, parallel to the shoulders, and the body is in the standing position. The hands should assume an overhand grip, a little more than shoulder-width apart. The arms are fully flexed at the elbows as the elbows point directly down to the floor. From this position the jerk and the overhead press movements are started.

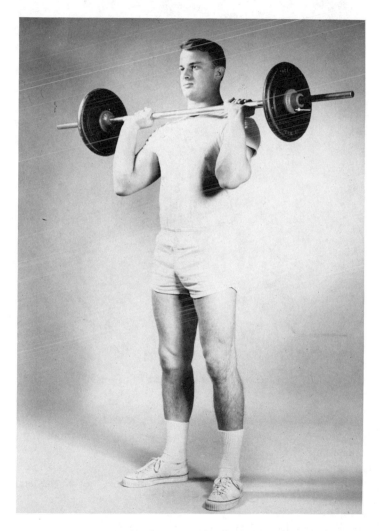

Figure 21. Chest-rest Position

5. Shoulder Rest — The bar is held across the back of the neck and shoulders, the body in the standing position. The overhand grip is used with the hands slightly more than shoulder width apart. As in the chest-rest position, the

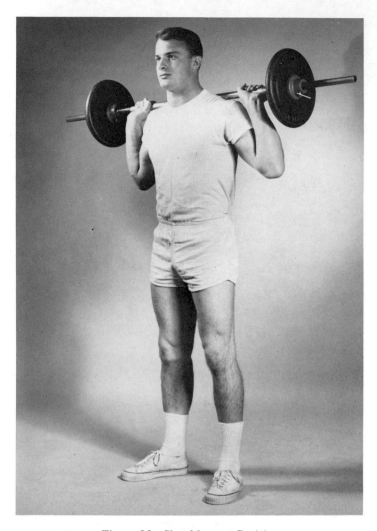

Figure 22. Shoulder-rest Position

arms are fully flexed with the elbows pointed directly to the floor. The barbell may be put into the shoulder rest position by spotters or by standing up from beneath a rack or frame used to hold the bar.

    6. Prone — This position is lying stretched out on the stomach.

    7. Supine — The opposite of prone; lying stretched out on the back.

DESCRIPTION OF WEIGHT-TRAINING EXERCISES

    Three divisions of exercises are described and illustrated: (1) the power-type exercise which increases overall strength and speed, (2) the basic strength-type exercise for specific use, and (3) power rack isometric exercises for alternate days and special work. Because power-type exercises are not included in many lifting programs, perhaps some additional explanation of their importance is needed.

Basic exercises for each muscle group are a definite part of the program, but putting different muscle groups together into one forceful action is also an invaluable part of weight training. In fact, power-type exercises are the very heart of weight training for athletes! These combination exercises closely resemble the powerful movement practiced in most sports. In their execution, equal emphasis should be placed on speed and strength.

Power is the most desirable quality an athlete can possess. For this reason the ultimate objective of weight training should be power improvement. The basic exercises are not sufficient by themselves because their final goal is strength and endurance in a particular muscle group, with some increase in power being only a by-product. As commonly practiced no special emphasis is placed on that other factor of power, speed. Those exercises which substantially increase power must combine the strength and speed overloads.

The training programs listed throughout this book incorporate two ideas that may deviate somewhat from standard weight-training programs. First, the two-set program of ten, and maximum repetitions recommended in this book is based on the idea that the first set performed with lighter weights can be devoted to speed-type lifting in which a powerful thrust can be executed. The power-type contractions should also be emphasized in the second set of repetitions, but the weight is usually too heavy for thrusting rapidly to position. The three-set program suggested for heavy days follows the same principle.

Second, power-type exercises involving a combination of body movements are recommended for each weight-training program. Originality is not claimed for either of these ideas. The only claim made is that power as well as strength can be improved if an effort is made to train for both. Included in this chapter is a list and description of general exercises in which a combination of muscular movements are combined into one explosive body action. Basic strength-building exercises for major muscle groups are included, but it is not felt that a wide variety of exercises are necessary in training for athletics.

The isometric exercises on the power rack listed and described in group three are very basic. The athlete can later devise other exercises to fit his special needs or to alter the routine. However, the illustrated exercises involve the majority of the muscle groups used in athletics.

In performing the isometric lifts it will take several sessions to determine the maximum lift for each position. If the lift can be performed for more than seven seconds, the trainee should add more weight to the bar.

The following exercises are considered basic:

A. Power Exercises
   1. Squat jump
   2. Modified clean

       3. Power curl

       4. Power press

       5. Dumbbell swing

       6. High pull-up

       7. Knee-bend and shoulder press

B. Basic Exercises

Neck Exercises

       8. Isometric flexion

       9. Isometric extension

     10. Wrestler's bridge

Shoulder Exercises

     11. Overhead press

     12. Rowing

     13. Rowing upright

     14. Shoulder press

     15. Lateral raise, standing

Arm Exercises

     16. Two-arm curl

     17. Tricep

     18. Chinning

     19. Shoulder dip

     20. Wrist curl

     21. Reverse wrist curl

Chest Exercises

     22. Bench press

     23. Straight-arm pullover

     24. Lateral raise, supine

Back Exercises

     25. Dead lift, straight legs

Abdominal Exercises

     26. Sit-up

     27. Leg-raise

Leg Exercises

     28. Squat

     29. Dead lift

     30. Heel-raise

     31. Knee flexor

     32. Knee extensor

C. Power Rack Isometric Exercises
    33. Isometric curl
    34. Isometric overhead press
    35. Isometric upright rowing
    36. Isometric dead lift
    37. Isometric bench press
    38. Isometric heel-raise

Figure 23. Skeletal Muscles, Front

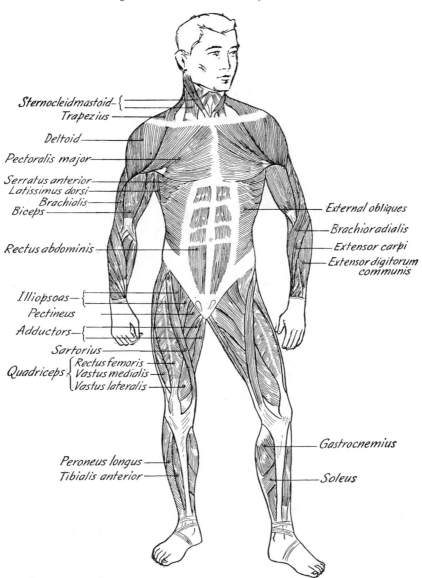

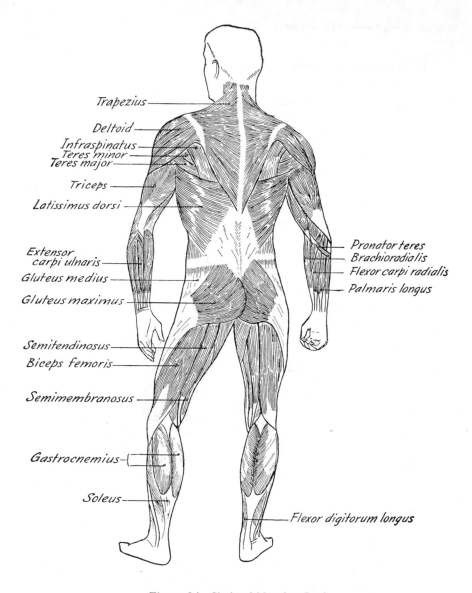

Trapezius

Deltoid

Infraspinatus
Teres minor
Teres major

Triceps

Latissimus dorsi

Extensor
carpi ulnaris

Gluteus medius

Gluteus maximus

Semitendinosus

Biceps femoris

Semimembranosus

Gastrocnemius-{

Soleus

Pronator teres
Brachioradialis
Flexor carpi radialis
Palmaris longus

Flexor digitorum longus

Figure 24. Skeletal Muscles, Back

Power Exercises

1. Squat jump

Equipment	Part Exercised	Primary Muscles
Dumbbells	Lower leg extensors	Quadriceps
	Thigh extensors	Gluteus Maximus
	Back extensors	Sacrospinalis

74

Hold a dumbbell in each hand and lower the body to a squat position with one foot advanced in front of the other. The legs and trunk are extended forcefully until they are completely straight and the feet are clear of the floor. While the body is in the air, the feet are reversed so that the leading foot in the first squat becomes the trailing foot in the second. Repeat this as many times as desired, alternating the feet each time. This is a vigorous leg and trunk exercise. The player should strive to jump as high as possible, springing from the balls of the feet and getting the head and shoulders back on each jump.

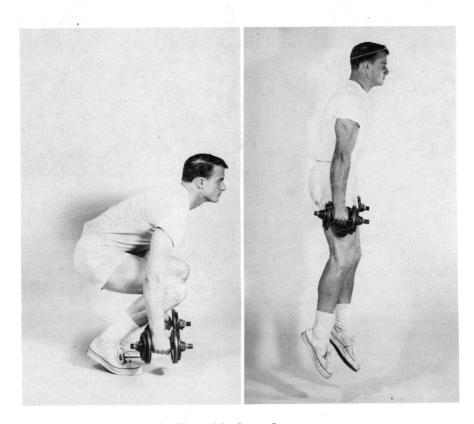

Figure 25. Squat Jump

2. **Modified clean**

Equipment	Part Exercised	Primary Muscles
Barbell	Lower leg extensors	Quadriceps
	Thigh extensors	Gluteus Maximus
	Arm flexors	Biceps
	Shoulder abductors	Deltoid

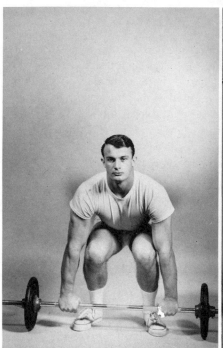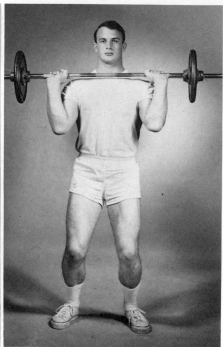

Figure 26. Modified Clean

From the crouch position, using an overhand grip, lift the bar with a very fast pull from the floor, employing the legs and hips until the legs are straight. At this point the bar should have acquired momentum. As the body straightens, the upward pull of the bar is continued by rising on the toes and pulling with the arms, keeping the bar close to the legs and body. When the bar reaches shoulder level the player dips under it with all of the speed possible to a half-squat. This action momentarily takes the weight off the wrists, enabling him to turn the wrists under and get his chest beneath the bar. It is important that the wrist and elbows be thrust under rapidly in order to better support the bar as it is brought to the chest and shoulders. The bar should travel from floor to shoulder-level in one continuous movement. After the bar is in this proper position the knees are straightened and the player stands erect. Return the bar to the starting position and repeat. This is an excellent explosive-type exercise to develop general body power.

3. **Power curl**

Equipment	Part Exercised	Primary Muscles
Barbell	Lower leg extensors	Quadriceps
	Thigh extensors	Gluteus Maximus
	Arm flexors	Biceps

Take a crouch position and grasp the bar with the hands shoulder-width apart, using an underhand grip. Curl the bar to the chest and stand to an erect position in one continuous motion. The muscles of the shoulders and back assist the biceps in bringing the bar to the chest at the fastest speed possible. Return the bar in the same arc to the starting position and repeat. The head and shoulders should be held back to prevent undue back strain. Much more weight should be used in this exercise than in the two-arm curl.

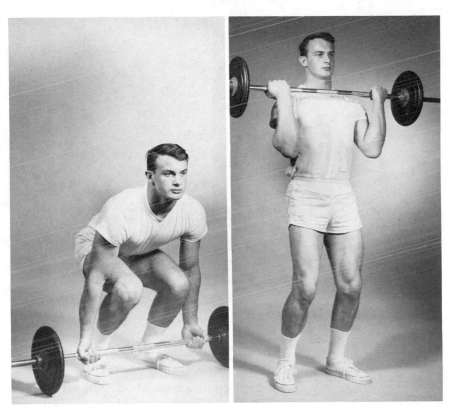

Figure 27. Power Curl

4. **Power press**

Equipment	*Part Exercised*	*Primary Muscles*
Barbell	Lower leg extensors	Quadriceps
	Arm extensors	Triceps
	Shoulder flexors	Deltoid

Position the bar at the chest rest position, with the hands in an overhand grip and shoulder-width apart. The legs are bent slightly at the knees and hips.

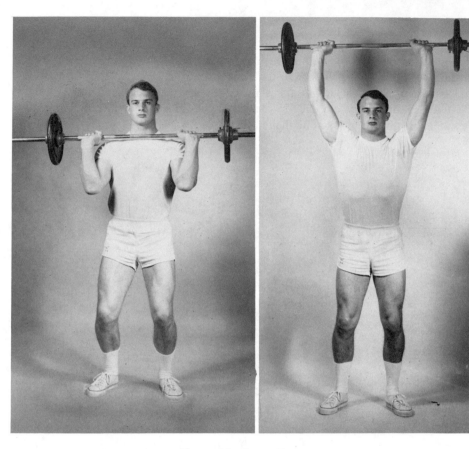

Figure 28. Power Press

Thrust the weight from the chest to an overhead position by straightening the legs and extending the arms. Return to the starting position and repeat. Use heavier weights than in the overhead press exercise and execute the thrusting movement with as much arm, shoulder, and leg force as can be brought into play.

5.   Dumbbell swing

Equipment	Part Exercised	Primary Muscles
Dumbbell	Arm extensors	Triceps
	Back extensors	Sacrospinalis

Load a dumbbell so that the plates are in the middle and room is left to grip the dumbbell on each end. Swing the weight overhead with both hands, allowing it to lower behind the neck as in the tricep exercise. The elbows should point straight up with the body erect and the legs spread wider than shoulder-width. Extend the arms forcefully overhead, swinging the dumbbell in a large arc until it goes between the legs in a chopping motion. Maintain its momentum and return it in the same arc to the starting position. The arms should extend fully overhead before the swinging motion begins. Allow the weight of the dumbbell to fully stretch the muscles of the back.

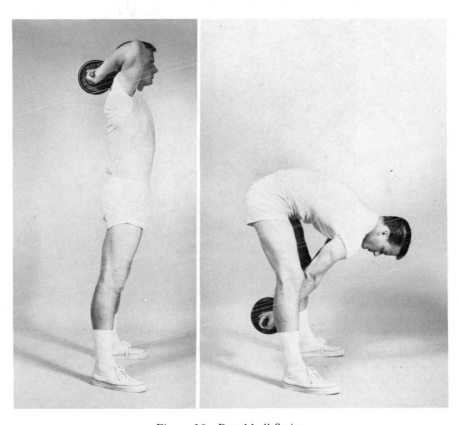

Figure 29. Dumbbell Swing

6. **High pull-up**

Equipment	Part Exercised	Primary Muscles
Barbell	Lower leg extensors	Quadriceps
	Thigh extensors	Gluteus Maximus
	Back extensors	Sacrospinalis
	Shoulder abductors	Deltoid
	Arm flexors	Biceps

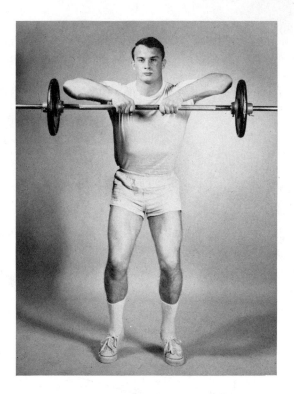

Figure 30. High Pull-up

Take a crouch position and grasp the bar with the hands about 6 inches apart, using an overhand grip. The arms should be positioned between the legs. Straightening the head and the back vigorously, stand erect and pull the bar up to the chin in one continuous motion. The elbows should remain higher than the hands throughout. Lower the barbell to the floor and repeat.

7. Knee-bend and shoulder press

Equipment	Part Exercised	Primary Muscles
Barbell	Lower leg extensors	Quadriceps
	Thigh extensors	Gluteus Maximus
	Shoulder abductors	Deltoid
	Arm extensors	Triceps

Place the barbell in a shoulder-rest position. Lower the body to a deep squat and come up forcefully, pushing the bar to a full overhead position in the same motion. Lower the bar again to the shoulder-rest position and repeat.

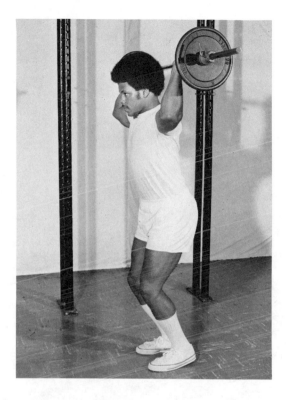

Figure 31. Knee-bend and Shoulder Press

Neck Exercises

8. **Isometric flexion**

Equipment	Part Exercised	Primary Muscles
None	Flexors	Sternomastoid
		Scaleni muscles
		Prevertebral muscles

Two players work together to perform this exercise. One positions himself on his hands and knees as the assistant cups his hands under the exerciser's forehead. The exerciser then exerts a downward force with his forehead against the assistant's hands for seven seconds. Three repetitions are executed. This exercise can be done alone by placing one's hands against the forehead and resisting the forehead flexion for seven seconds. In organized programs, however, it is more effective to work in pairs.

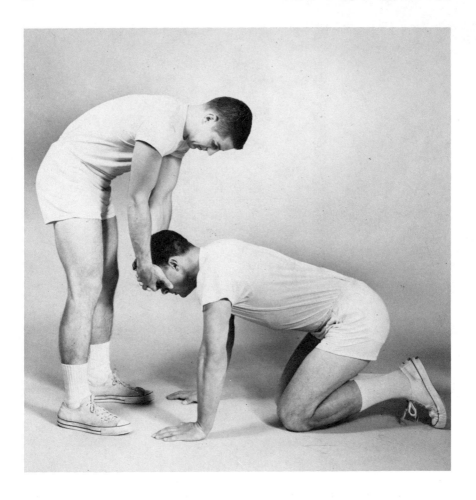

Figure 32. Isometric Flexion

9. Isometric extension

Equipment	Part Exercised	Primary Muscles
None	Extensors	Sacrospinalis
		Splenius
		Semispinalis
		Deep posterior spinal muscles

   The players work together as in the isometric flexion exercises, assuming the same relative positions. The assistant places his hands on the back of the exerciser's head and resists for seven seconds his efforts to lift it. Three repetitions are executed. The assistant should lock his elbows and only resist the isometric exercise. He should not push down. After two or three weeks it is suggested that the exerciser attempt to push his head up, right and left. This exercise can also be performed alone by interlocking the fingers and placing the hands behind the head, resisting the forehead extension for six seconds.

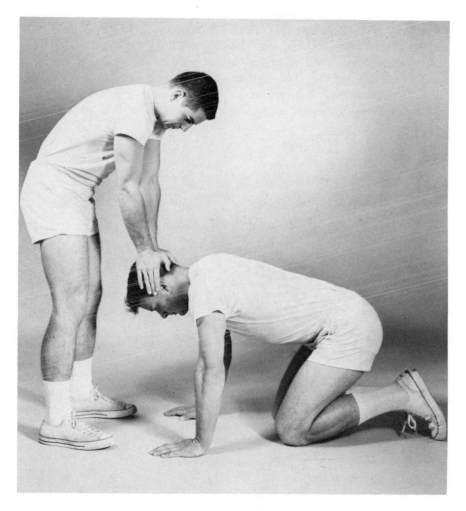

Figure 33. Isometric Extension

Isometric exercises are not usually considered for weight-training routines, but the isometric neck exercises can be more easily included in an organized program than other more conventional ones, and have proven very effective.

10. Wrestler's bridge

Equipment	*Part Exercised*	*Primary Muscles*
Weight	Flexors and extensors	Same as Exercises 8 and 9

Take supine position with the head on a mat or some other soft surface. Bend the knees and place the feet flat on the floor, close to the buttocks. Hold the hands across the chest and raise the body off the floor by arching the neck and back and pushing with the legs. The full body weight should be supported by the head and the feet. The exercise can be made more difficult by rocking back and forth and by holding a weight on the chest. A beginner should work with the isometric exercises for several weeks before undertaking the wrestler's bridge.

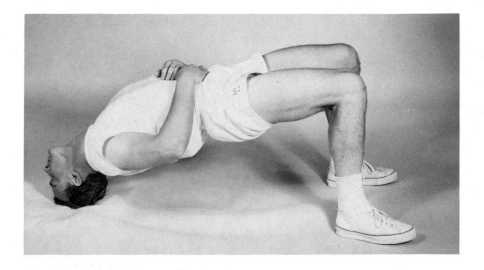

Figure 34. Wrestler's Bridge

Shoulder Exercises

11. Overhead press

Equipment	*Part Exercised*	*Primary Muscles*
Barbell	Abductors	Deltoid
	Flexors	Coracobrachialis
	Arm extensors	Triceps

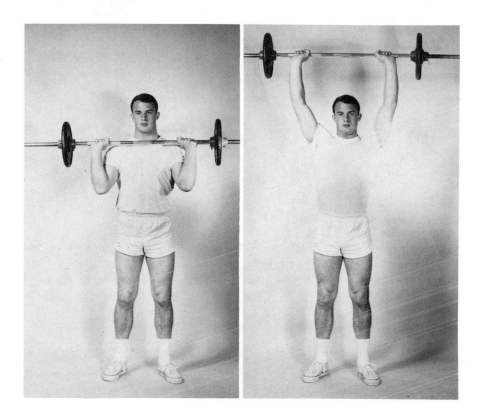

Figure 35. Overhead Press

Clean the bar to the chest-rest position. The feet should be comfortably positioned about shoulder-width apart. Push the weight from the shoulders to an overhead position, locking the arms at the elbows. Do not bend the knees or lean back to an unnatural position in the process of pressing the bar. Lower the bar to the chest-rest position and repeat.

12. Rowing

Equipment	Part Exercised	Primary Muscles
Barbell	Extensors	Latissimus Dorsi
		Teres Major
	Arm flexors	Brachialis

Stand with the feet a comfortable distance apart and bend from the hips ɔ a position where the upper body is parallel with the floor. The knees should

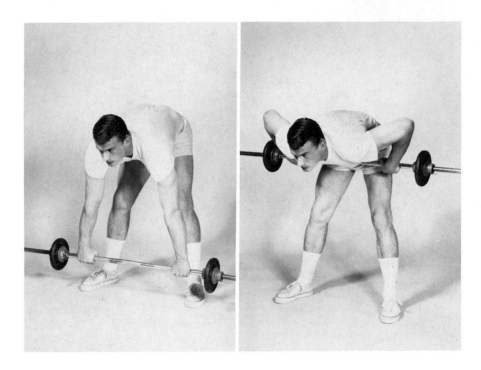

Figure 36. Rowing

be bent slightly. Grasp the bar with an overhand grip slightly more than shoulder-width apart. Pull the bar to the body at the upper abdomen. Lower the bar to an arm-hang position and repeat. Do not let the bar touch the floor between repetitions. It is especially important that a beginner bend the knees slightly during this exercise in order to reduce tension on the lower back.

13. Rowing upright

Equipment	Part Exercised	Primary Muscles
Barbell	Abductors	Deltoid
		Supraspinatus
	Arm flexors	Biceps

Using an overhand grip, grasp the bar in the center with the hands about 6 inches apart. Stand erect, letting the bar hang at a thigh-rest position. Pull the bar up to the chin, keeping the elbows higher than the hands throughout. Lower the bar to the starting position and repeat the movement. Only the arms and shoulders should move during this exercise.

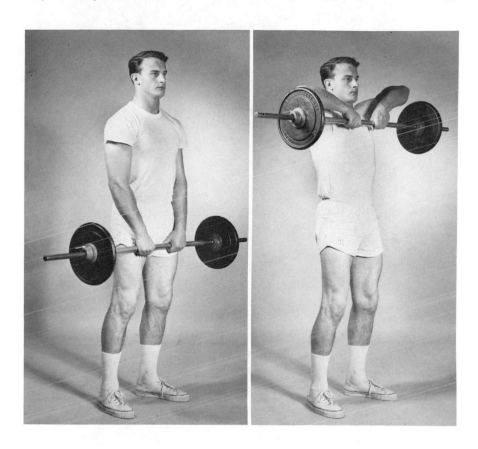

Figure 37. Rowing Upright

14. Shoulder press

Barbell	*Part Exercised*	*Primary Muscles*
	Abductors	Deltoid
		Supraspinatus
	Arm extensors	Triceps

Using an overhand grip, grasp the bar with hands spaced wider than shoulder-width. Clean and press the bar, positioning it at the shoulder-rest position well down on the shoulders. Press the bar from this position to a full-arms extension, and return to the starting position. Repeat for the desired number of repetitions, remembering to keep the head bent forward slightly to avoid contact with the bar.

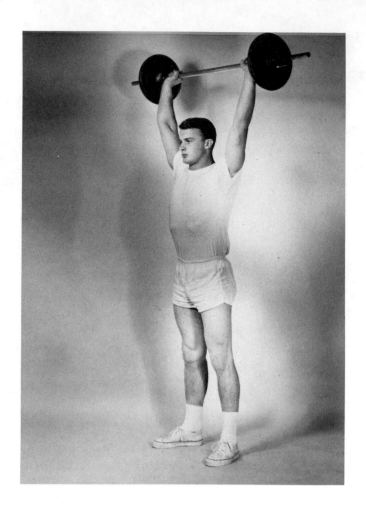

Figure 38. Shoulder Press

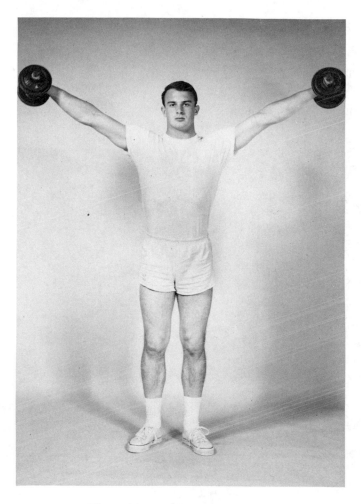

Figure 39. Lateral Raise, Standing

15. Lateral raise, standing

Equipment	*Part Exercised*	*Primary Muscles*
Dumbbells	Abductors	Deltoid
		Supraspinatus

Stand with the feet comfortably spaced, the hands holding a dumbbell at each side, the palms facing the body. Raise the dumbbells directly sideways to head-level position, keeping the arms straight throughout. Lower to the starting osition and repeat.

Arm Exercises

16. Two-arm curl

Equipment	Part Exercised	Primary Muscles
Barbell	Flexors	Biceps
		Brachialis

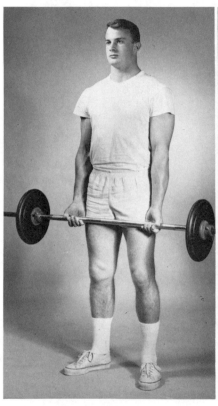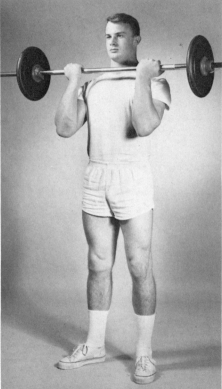

Figure 40. Two-arm Curl

Using an underhand grip, grasp the bar with the hands shoulder-width apart. Stand erect, the bar hanging at a thigh rest position. The feet should be comfortably spread. Keeping the upper arms motionless and close to the body, flex the arms at the elbow joint until the bar touches the chest. Return the bar in the same arc to the starting position and repeat.

17. Tricep

Equipment	Part Exercised	Primary Muscles
Barbell	Extensors	Triceps

Using an overhand grip, grasp the bar with the hands spaced no more than 10 inches apart. Clean and press the bar, positioning it across the back of the neck and shoulders. The elbows should point directly up. From this position press the bar to a full overhead extension and return to the starting position. Keep the head bent slightly forward to avoid contacting the bar.

Figure 41. Tricep

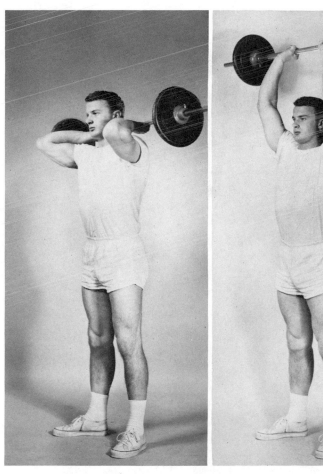
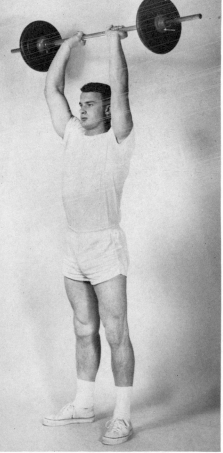

18. Chinning

Equipment	Part Exercised	Primary Muscles
Chinning bar	Flexors	Biceps
		Brachialis
	Shoulder extensor	Latissimus Dorsi

Grasp the chinning bar using an underhand grip. From a full-arm extension position pull the body up to a position at which the chin is above the bar. Return to the original position and repeat. When the exercise can be repeated ten times, add to the weight of the body by tying a weight plate around the neck. Caution the player to reach a full arm extension after each pull-up.

Figure 42. Chinning

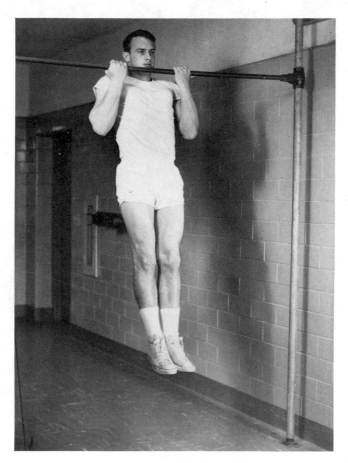

19. Shoulder dip

Equipment	Part Exercised	Primary Muscles
Parallel bars	Extensors	Triceps

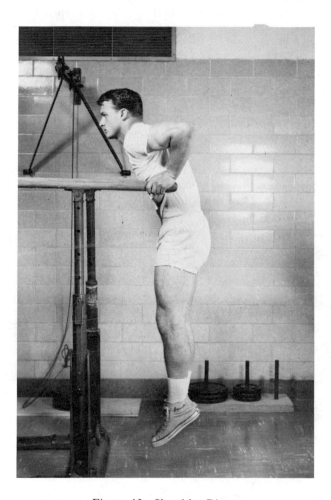

Figure 43. Shoulder Dip

Assume a position at the end of the parallel bars which has the body hanging between them, supported by the hands and arms. The arms are at the sides and locked at the elbows. Allow the body to dip between the bars by bending the arms at the elbows. When the upper arms come to a position parallel to the bars, extend the arms and return to the original position.

Forearm Exercises

20. Wrist curl

Equipment	*Part Exercised*	*Primary Muscles*
Barbell	Flexors	Flexor Carpi muscles

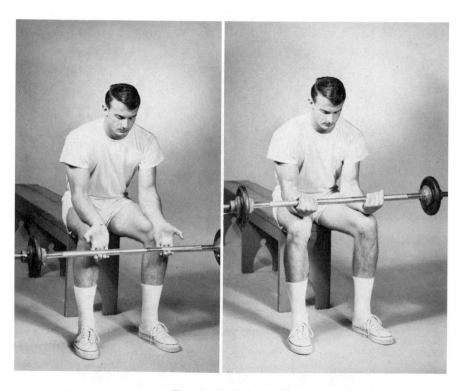

Figure 44. Wrist Curl

Grasp the bar, using an underhand grip, and sit on the exercise bench. The feet should be flat on the floor with the forearms resting on the thighs. Extend the wrists, allowing the bar to roll as far as possible toward the fingertips. The fingers and wrists are then flexed to a maximum contraction of the forearm and finger flexor muscles. Only enough grip is maintained to prevent the bar from slipping from the grasp. Allow the bar to roll back down the fingers and return in the same arc. Repeat.

21. Reverse wrist curl

Equipment	*Part Exercised*	*Primary Muscles*
Barbell	Extensors	Extensor Carpi muscles

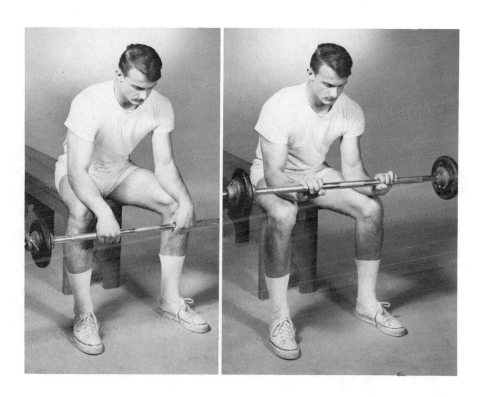

Figure 45. Reverse Wrist Curl

Grasp the bar, using an overhand grip, and sit on the exercise bench. Again position the feet flat on the floor with the forearms resting on the thighs. Allow the weight of the bar to carry the wrist to a fully flexed position, the weight being supported by the thumb and the ends of the fingers. Raise the bar in an arc by contracting the extensor muscles of the forearm, keeping the forearms resting on the thighs. Allow the bar to return in the same arc and repeat.

Chest Exercises

22. **Bench press**

Equipment	Part Exercised	Primary Muscles
Barbell	Shoulder horizontal flexors	Anterior Deltoid
		Pectoralis Major
	Arm extensors	Triceps

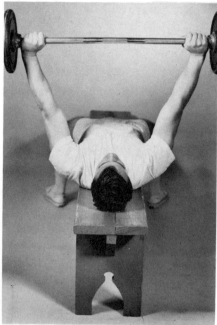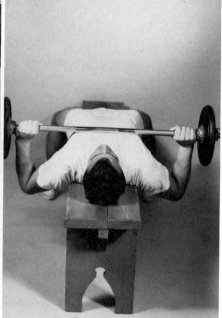

Figure 46. Bench Press

Assume a supine position on the bench with the head, shoulders, and hips contacting it and the legs straddling it, feet flat on the floor. Take the barbell off the rack or from two assistants in a straight-arm supporting position. Use an overhand grip and grasp the barbell slightly wider than shoulder-width. Lower the bar to the chest and press it to the straight-arm position as many times as desired. No body motion is permitted, so refrain from bridging the buttocks off the bench during the press. Inhale while pressing and exhale as the arms are locked. Holding the elbows wide will bring the pectoral muscles into greater use.

23. Straight-arm pullover

Equipment	Part Exercised	Primary Muscles
Barbell	Shoulder extensors	Deltoid
		Pectoralis Major
		Teres Major
		Latissimus Dorsi
		Triceps

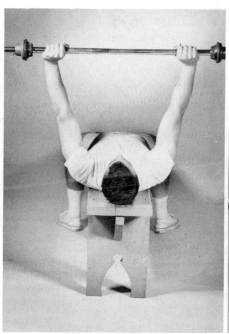 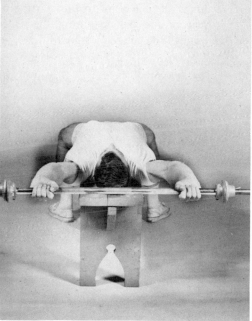

Figure 47. Straight-arm Pullover

Lie supine on the mat or bench and hold the barbell at a full arm-extension position over the chest. The overhand grip is used and the hands are spaced slightly wider than shoulder-width. Keeping the arms straight, lower the bar in an arc to a position directly above the head and, after a brief pause, return it in the same arc. Inhale deeply during the first movement and exhale as the bar is returned to its original position. The weight of the bar is usually as much as a beginner should use in this exercise. Strive for correct breathing.

24. Lateral raise, supine

Equipment	Part Exercised	Primary Muscles
Dumbbells	Shoulder horizontal flexors	Anterior Deltoid
		Pectoralis Major
		Coracobrachialis

While supine on an exercise bench, hold a pair of dumbbells directly over the chest with the palms of the hands facing in. Bend the arms slightly and keep them bent throughout the exercise. Lower the weights in an arc to the sides and return in the same arc to the starting position. Inhale deeply during the first movement and exhale during the second. The exercise may be varied by practicing it on an inclined board.

Figure 48. Lateral Raise, Supine

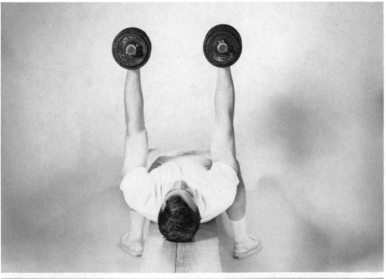
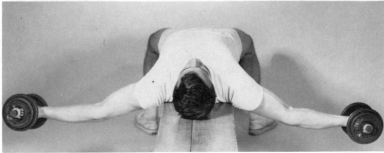

Back Exercises

25. Dead lift, straight legs

Equipment	Part Exercised	Primary Muscles
Barbell	Back extensors	Sacrospinalis
	Hip extensors	Gluteus Maximus

Grasp the bar with the hands about shoulder-width apart, using the overhand grip, and lift it to a thigh-rest position. Lower the weight to the floor by bending at the hips, keeping the knees fully extended so that the posterior leg muscles will be stretched. Return to the thigh-rest position and repeat. The arms and hands should hang straight throughout the exercise. In reality, this is a toe-touching exercise with the bar. No attempt should be made to progress to exceptionally heavy weights with this exercise. Beginners should start with no more than 40 or 50 pounds.

Figure 49. Dead Lift, Straight Legs

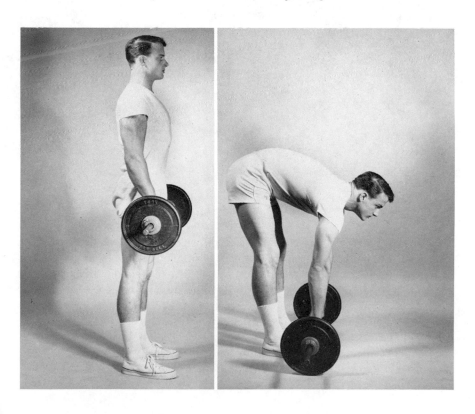

Abdominal Exercises

26. **Sit-up**

Equipment	*Part Exercised*	*Primary Muscles*
Weight	Flexors	Rectus Abdominis
		Obliques
	Hip flexors	Psoas Major

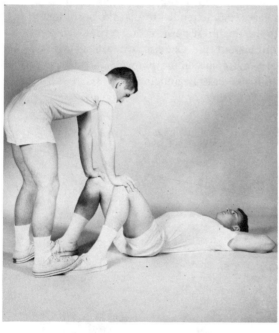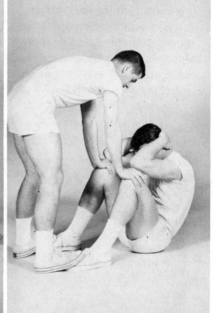

Figure 50. Sit-up

In a supine position, place the feet and ankles under a loaded barbell or have a partner hold the feet in a stationary position. Lock the hands behind the head and curl to a sitting position. Curl the head first, then the shoulders, then the back. Lower yourself back to the original position touching the lower back, the shoulders, and the head in the order named. As abdominal strength improves the exercise should be made more difficult by performing it with feet flat on the floor and knees bent, and later by holding a weight behind the head.

An excellent variation is curling only halfway up and holding for five seconds before lowering to the original position.

27. Leg-raise

Equipment	Part Exercised	Primary Muscles
None	Hip flexors	Iliopsoas
	Trunk flexors	Rectus Abdominis
	Leg extensors	Quadriceps

Lie in a supine position with the hands under the head and the back flattened against the floor. Point the toes and lift the legs off the floor to a verticle position, keeping them as straight as possible. Lower them to the floor, touching only briefly with the heels, and repeat the desired number of times.

Figure 51. Leg-raise

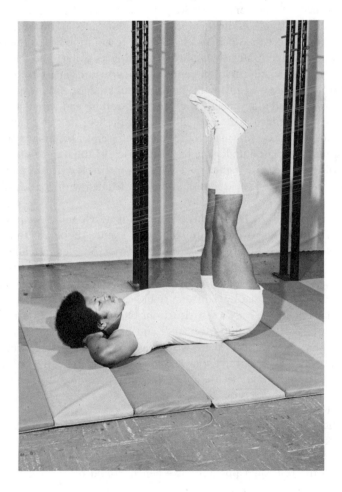

Leg Exercises

28. **Squat**

Equipment	*Part Exercised*	*Primary Muscles*
Barbell	Thigh extensors	Gluteus Maximus
	Lower leg extensors	Quadriceps

Start with relatively light weights during the learning stages. The bar should rest across the shoulders and back of the neck with the hands grasping it at somewhat greater than shoulder-width apart. The exerciser puts the bar in position by executing a clean and press and lowering the bar to the shoulders behind the neck. When very heavy weights are desired it becomes necessary to have two assistants place the bar across the shoulders. Many weight-training rooms are equipped with squat racks or stands to hold the bar so the trainer has only to stoop under it slightly to be in a lifting position. The feet should be comfortably positioned, usually about shoulder-width apart with the heels elevated on a two-inch board. With the back kept straight and the chest high the body is lowered into a three-quarter squat position and raised to a starting position as many times as desired, inhaling as the legs flex and exhaling while they extend. Beginners will need to be cautioned against bending at the waist. A small pad may be placed under the bar at the back of the trainee's neck. Greater balance will be called for if the squat is done on the toes. This is more difficult than the heel-supported squat and should be performed with comparatively light weights.

The squat exercise is probably the best for development of powerful legs and hips. There is controversy as to whether a trainer should go to a full squat position with heavy weight because of the danger of overstretching the knee stabilizers. It should be said that there are many weight trainers who perform the full squat with no deleterious effects. However, some others have a great deal of difficulty, probably caused by a difference in anatomical structure.

Actually there are only a few situations in modern sports in which a player is called on to perform a full knee-bend, and because there is apparently some danger of injury to the knee, there is no reason for an athlete to train with the full squat exercise. The three-quarter squat will exercise the same muscles equally as well and eliminate the injury hazard. Therefore, in references to the squat or knee-bend exercise throughout this book the reference is to the three-quarter squat.

If there is difficulty stopping at the three-quarter squat position (with the thighs approximately parallel to the floor) a good precaution is to place a low bench behind the legs so that the trainee will sit on the bench rather than continue to the full squat position. The bench should be an inch or two lower than the knees.

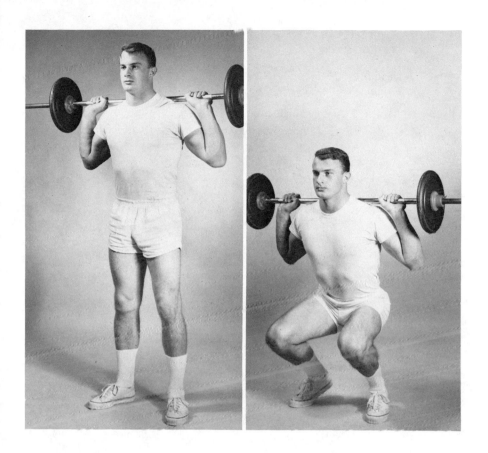

Figure 52. Squat

29. Dead lift

Equipment	Part Exercised	Primary Muscles
Barbell	Thigh extensors	Gluteus Maximus
	Lower leg extensors	Quadriceps
	Back extensors	Sacrospinalis

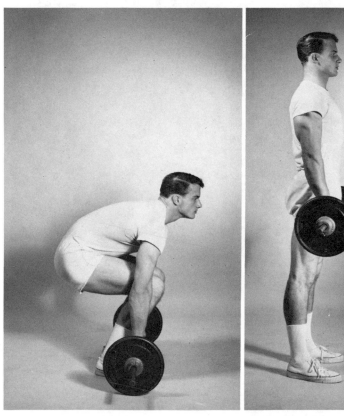
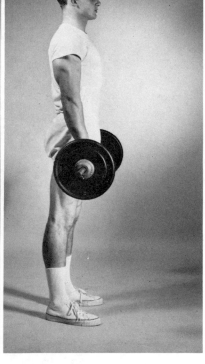

Figure 53. Dead Lift

Assume a crouch position with the head up and the back straight. Grasp the barbell with the hands shoulder-width apart, using an overhand grip. Keeping the shoulders back and the chest high, stand up to an erect position, lifting the barbell to a thigh-rest position. Keeping the arms straight throughout the exercise, lower to the starting position and repeat. Inhale while lifting and exhale while returning to the starting position.

30. Heel-raise

Equipment	Part Exercised	Primary Muscles
Barbell	Foot plantar flexors	Gastrocnemius
		Soleus

Place the barbell across the back of the neck and shoulders, the hands grasping the bar at slightly more than shoulder-width. Place the toes on a 2- to 3-inch board and raise forcefully to full height on the toes. Lower to the original position and repeat. Position the feet so the toes point out, in, and straight ahead to vary the exercise. The heel-raises should be performed with a powerful movement for best results and because the calves need a large amount of work it is best to do as many as ten to twelve repetitions at each toe position.

Figure 54. Heel-raise

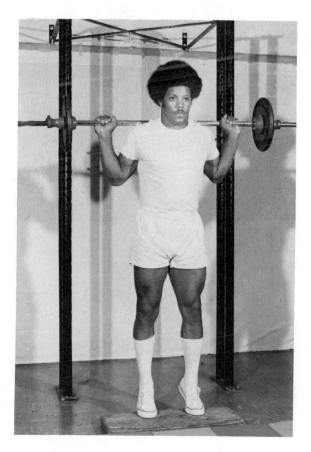

31. Knee flexor

Equipment	Part Exercised	Primary Muscles
Iron boot	Flexors	Hamstrings

Attach an iron boot to one foot and stand on the exercise bench, allowing the weighted foot to hang over the edge. Hold the wall for support. Perform the exercise by flexing the knee as much as possible while maintaining the hip in an extended position. Lower yourself slowly to the starting position and repeat for the desired number of times before exercising the other leg. The hip flexors may be exercised by lifting the thigh up high and allowing the knee to flex passively.

Figure 55. Knee Flexor

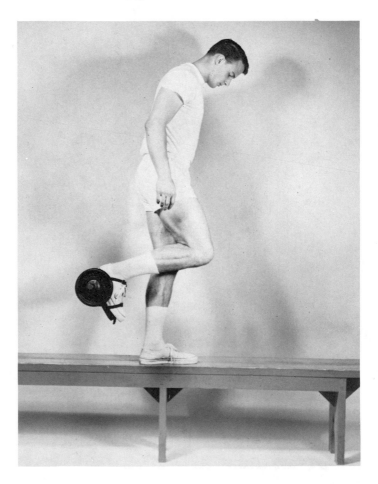

32. Knee extensor

Equipment	Part Exercised	Primary Muscles
Iron boot	Extensors	Quadriceps

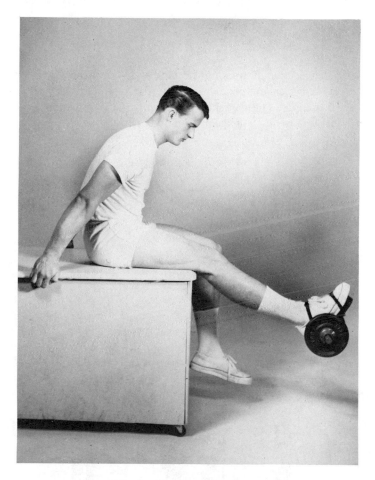

Figure 56. Knee Extensor

Again an iron boot is attached to one foot as the trainee sits on the end of a table, with the legs supported from hip to knee by the table. The boot is raised in an arc until the knee is fully extended. Let the boot return slowly to the starting position and repeat for the desired number of times before exercising the other leg.

Power Rack Isometric Exercises

33.   Isometric curl

Equipment	Part Exercised	Primary Muscles
Power rack	Arm flexors	Biceps
		Brachialis

Set the bar so that it rests on the pins at approximately belt-level when standing erect. Using an underhand grip, lift the bar and hold against the top pins for seven seconds. The feet should be comfortably spread and the elbows should be kept close to, but not against the body.

Figure 57. Isometric Curl

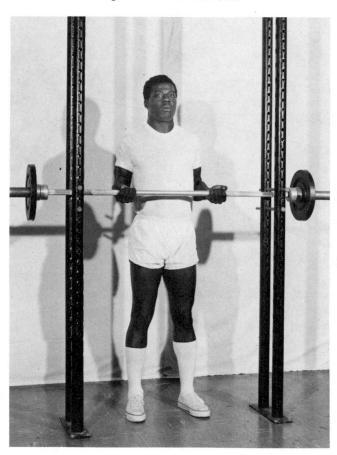

34. Isometric overhead press

Equipment	Part Exercised	Primary Muscles
Power rack	Shoulder flexors	Deltoid
	Arm extensors	Coracobrachialis
		Triceps

Set the bar so that it barely clears the top of the head when standing erect. Stand under and slightly behind the bar. The hands and feet should be approximately a shoulder-width apart. Press the bar against the top pins for seven seconds, being careful not to lean back to an unnatural position in the process of pressing the bar.

Figure 58. Isometric Overhead Press

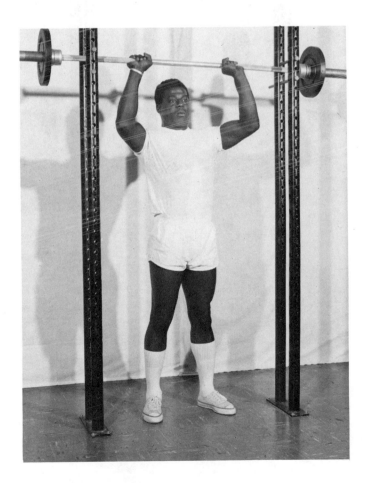

35. Isometric upright rowing

Equipment	Part Exercised	Primary Muscles
Power rack	Shoulder abductors	Deltoid
	Arm flexors	Supraspinatus
		Biceps
		Trapezius

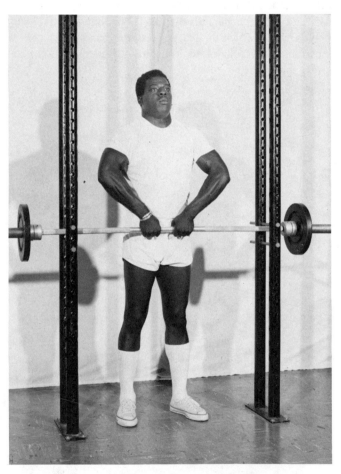

Figure 59. Isometric Upright Rowing

Set the pins so that the bar strikes the trainee, when standing erect, at a point approximately four inches below the waist. Using an overhand grip, grasp the bar in the center with the hands about six inches apart. Pull the bar up against the top pins, keeping the elbows away from the body and pointed out. The effort should be with the shoulders as well as the arm flexors.

36.   Isometric dead lift

Equipment	Part Exercised	Primary Muscles
Power rack	Thigh extensors	Gluteus maximus
	Lower leg extensors	Quadriceps
	Back extensors	Sacrospinalis

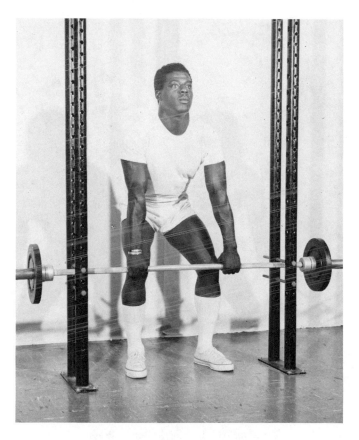

Figure 60. Isometric Dead Lift

Set the pins so that when the proper exercise position is assumed the bar strikes the lifter across the thighs about three or four inches above the knee. The knee angle should be about 135 degrees. Assume a position with the head up and the back straight. Grasp the bar with an overhand grip, keeping the hands about shoulder-width apart. The feet are also about shoulder-width apart with the insteps of the feet directly under the bar. Lift the bar against the top pins, using the leg and back muscles and using the arms only to hold the bar.

37. Isometric bench press

Equipment	Part Exercised	Primary Muscles
Power rack	Shoulder horizontal flexors	Anterior deltoid
		Pectoralis major
	Arm extensors	Triceps

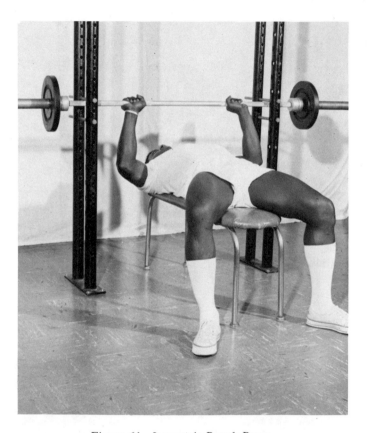

Figure 61. Isometric Bench Press

Place a bench under the bar and assume a supine position on the bench so that the bar is directly over the chest. The head, shoulders, and hips should contact the bench and the legs should straddle it, with the feet flat on the floor. Use an overhand grip and grasp the bar slightly wider than shoulder-width. The bar should be set high enough so that when the force is applied and the bar is lifted against the top pins, the arms at the elbow joint are at approximately a 90-degree angle. No body motion is indicated.

38. Isometric heel raise

Equipment	Part Exercised	Primary Muscles
Power rack	Foot plantar flexors	Gastrocnemius
		Soleus

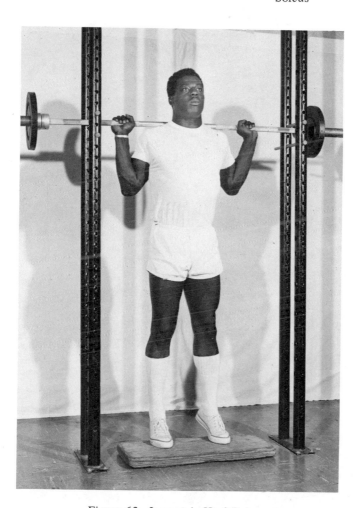

Figure 62. Isometric Heel Raise

Set the pins so that the bar is barely above the shoulders. Place a pad or doubled towel on the shoulders. Grasp the bar so that the hands are slightly more than shoulder-width apart. Raise forcefully by standing on the toes, pushing the bar against the top pins with the shoulders.

6

WEIGHT TRAINING
IN BASEBALL

The muscle-boundness myth has prevailed in baseball probably more than in any other sport. Until recent years there has been a peculiar but widely accepted theory that a baseball player who dares to touch a barbell will become so tight in the arms and shoulders that he will lose the skill and coordination required to perform the unique baseball skills of hitting and throwing. As previously discussed, clinical evidence has not supported such a theory. On the contrary it has revealed that such a theory is based on ignorance and hearsay.

If two boys have the same degree of skill in playing baseball, the stronger one has a much better chance to succeed. Experiments we have conducted over the years have shown conclusively that not only is there a very high correlation between strength and success in hitting and throwing a baseball, but there is a definite improvement in the ability of the individual when his strength is noticeably increased.

In one experiment[1] involving more than fifty college freshmen we measured ability in hitting and throwing for distance and measured with an aircraft tensiometer the strength of the same individuals in the shoulder, arm, and hand areas. An examination of the most pertinent correlations revealed that in this study a very high correlation existed between shoulder strength and hitting and throwing, and a moderately high correlation existed between forearm strength and these two baseball skills. The relation between grip strength and the two skills was significant but not nearly so significant as the other body areas mentioned. Strength in the hands is certainly an important factor but it has apparently been vastly overrated.

[1]G. E. Hooks, "The Effect of Weight Training on the Baseball Skills of Hitting, Running, and Throwing" (unpublished study). Wake Forest College, 1958.

Assuming that there is a close relation between strength and baseball ability, what is the best way to acquire this strength? Various theories have been discussed previously. Ty Cobb ran in weighted shoes. Johnny Mize reportedly spent the winter chopping wood. Some major league stars have trained with weights. In each of these methods of strength-training the physiological effect is similar. The muscle must work against resistance to improve. It must be overloaded.

For many years the conditioning program of a baseball player has been to run and run and run. The slogan, "Get those legs in shape and you won't have a sore arm," has been the pivotal point around which the majority of baseball conditioning programs have functioned. Perhaps the logic behind this program was good when the average player was brought up in an environment involving exposure to substantial amounts of manual labor with hands and arms. A conditioning program for such a player would best be a program of running and stretching exercises. But today's player does not ordinarily get the necessary hand and arm exercises from his environment.

Most baseball coaches have trained teams by giving them large doses of hitting and throwing to supplement the running program. Granted it is impossible to get in condition for baseball without much practice in these skills; but it should be noted that players lift nothing heavier than a ball, a bat, and a glove. This certainly doesn't involve overloading the muscles, and it surely doesn't develop much strength, or the players wouldn't have to swing two or three bats in order to make one seem lighter. Mastery of the skills is not enough. Strength and power are needed to excel.

As has been indicated earlier, ours is a mechanized age. The times have changed but baseball rules have not. The youth of today have a much better opportunity to play baseball, and as a result are probably more skilled than their predecessors. However, they have much less opportunity to develop strength through manual labor. An untold number of well-skilled players with outstanding potential have not been successful because they lacked basic body strength, especially in the arms and shoulders. For this reason a program of baseball conditioning that pivots around progressive resistive exercise directed at improving strength and power in running, hitting, and throwing muscles seems imperative.

In another experiment[2] a group of thirty freshmen was tested on the baseball skills of hitting and throwing for distance. Their strength in the wrist, elbow, and shoulder joints was then measured. After completing the tests the group participated in a basic body-building program using weights. They were not allowed to practice either of the baseball skills. At the end of six weeks they were retested. The results revealed an improvement in strength, and even though the group did not at any time practice hitting and throwing for distance, they

[2]G. E. Hooks, "Prediction of Baseball Ability Through An Analysis of Measures of Strength and Structure," *Research Quarterly,* 30 (1959), 38–44.

showed a marked improvement in both of these skills. Throwing for distance revealed the greatest improvement. Only three of the thirty students failed to beat their previous scores in this test. The results of the other tests were less dramatic but they confirmed our belief that weight training can be used to advantage in baseball training.

Baseball capitalizes on sudden bursts of strength and power, but by its nature does little to develop them. Hitting, running, and throwing involve the vigorous action of many muscles for very brief periods. Running calls for quick bursts of speed. Hitting and throwing usually involve sudden and vigorous muscular contractions. The body must be properly conditioned for strength and endurance to avoid muscle strain and joint damage. This conditioning can best be accomplished through a program combining weight training, skill drills, and running.

Weight training has been used by many outstanding major league baseball players to build powerful arms for hitting and throwing. Usually they refrain from advertising it, either because their managers frown on the idea or because they don't wish others to have the same advantage. However, many other major leaguers have used weights to improve their strength and the indications are that there will be many more.

DISCUSSION OF SKILLS

The skills of hitting, throwing, fielding, and running are not entirely peculiar to baseball, but are certainly the primary criteria for measuring success. Other tangible assets, such as desire, depth perception, reflex action, etc., are essential as well, but the fundamental skills should be the primary interest of the coach. In this day of specialization it is possible for a player to master only one of the skills involved so long as he has better than average ability in the others. Some of the highest-salaried players are pinch hitters who aren't usually good enough to play regularly. Most pitchers in professional baseball are mediocre hitters, and some fielding whizzes are often inserted in the lineup for defensive purposes. Fast runners are used as pinch runners when a slow man gets on base.

The basic weight program recommended in Chapter 11 can be used to advantage with any baseball player, the results being improved strength, endurance, and ability to handle the body weight. Such a program combined with agility drills will be valuable for improving fielding ability. Specific exercises for fielding are not prescribed, however, so it is not discussed in detail. Running in baseball is very similar to that of track, and is described in detail in Chapter 10. Hitting and throwing can be significantly improved through weight training and are discussed below. Hitting and throwing techniques are described, and to help the reader set up a conditioning program a description of the muscular action for each skill has been included.

Hitting

Hitting is one of the more exacting baseball skills, requiring muscular strength and coordination for successful achievement. The variety of stances and mannerisms characterized by many of the game's greatest hitters make generalizations in regard to form and technique difficult. Basically speaking, however, the great hitters follow a pattern. The following discussion concerns right-handed hitters only; the analysis is reversed for left-handed hitters.

In the preparatory position the head should be turned in line with the shoulders, the eyes trained on the pitcher. The hands should be held close together, the arms keeping the bat in a ready position behind the right shoulder, the larger end of the bat well above the smaller end. The left elbow should be partially flexed, while the right elbow is flexed and pointed down. The bat is held firmly and far enough from the body to allow freedom of movement. The trunk should be fairly erect but relaxed, and should be rotated to the right. The knees should be slightly flexed with the feet spaced comfortably apart, generally perpendicular to a line from the pitcher to the plate. As the ball approaches, the batter should shift most of his weight to his rear foot.

As in the throw, the initial movement of the swing is the stride with the left foot. As the stride is started the arms and hips go into action. The large end of the bat is lowered to a level position and is swung forcefully with a straightening of the arms and a snap and roll of the wrists. In coordination with the arm action, the hips should rotate sharply to the left and the body weight should be pressed against a firm front leg by a strong drive with the rear leg. At the instant the bat contacts the ball the large end should be slightly ahead of the hands. The finish of the swing involves a follow-through of the body in the direction of the batted ball.

Hitting a baseball is a complicated movement in which one muscle group of the body functions exactly opposite to its counterpart. For example, when the right-handed hitter swings, the pronator of the right forearm contracts simultaneously with the supinator of the left forearm. A natural temptation is to concentrate on the development of the muscles that specifically control these movements. This is not practical, however, because it is imperative to maintain good muscular balance between opposite, or antagonistic, muscle groups.

The muscles of the shoulders (deltoid, infraspinatus, pectoralis major) are probably the most important in hitting a ball with power. They generate the initial force that gets the bat under way and give the smaller muscles of the arms and hands the strong foundation they need to contract maximally. The elbow extensors (triceps) continue the bat along its path and the muscles of the forearms (pronators and supinators) and hands (flexor and extensor carpi groups) provide the final impetus. It is imperative that the wrist flexors and extensors be developed to such a degree that they not only control the direction of the swing but can also deliver the final blow with maximum power.

The muscles of the trunk and legs provide the foundation for the swing. The hip extensors (gluteus maximus), knee extensors (quadriceps), and ankle plantar flexors (gastrocnemius, soleus) are a terrific driving force if the swing is timed properly, and they should be well-developed. The rotators of the hips (gluteus maximus and minimus) are also important and need specific exercise.

Throwing

The distance a ball may be thrown is dependent upon a coordinated movement of the entire body. The actions of the arms, hips, and legs must be brought into play at precisely the right instant for each to contribute to maximum distance.

The distance of the throw is directly related to the strength used in throwing the ball and to the speed of hand and fingers at the moment of release. Weakness in one of the participating muscle groups will cut down on the distance or the speed of the throw. The following discussion concerns right-handed throwers only; the analysis is reversed for left-handed throwers.

The preparatory position for throwing a ball is fairly typical. The ball should be held in such a manner that when the palm of the hand is down the first and second fingers are on top and slightly apart. The thumb furnishes pressure underneath, while the third and fourth fingers steady the ball on the right side. The ball should be held loosely in the fingers and toward the fingertips.

In the winding-up action of the body much depends upon the muscles of the trunk and lower limbs. The trunk is rotated far toward the right, extending the muscles responsible for the powerful contraction needed to begin the throw. The right arm carries the ball back above the level of the ear. In the wind-up position the elbow of the right arm is partially bent, the wrist is hyperextended, and the fingers grasp the ball firmly. The left arm is swung in front of the body to aid in balance. The left shoulder is held low to avoid interference with the thrower's vision.

The throwing motion is preceded by a long stride with the left foot and an accompanying shift in weight to that leg. As the left foot hits the ground in line with the target, the ball is thrown from the right shoulder with a strong pronated movement of the forearm. The flexor muscles of the wrist and fingers provide the final impetus. Whether the throw is overhand or sidearm, the elbow travels at a lower level than the ball and usually precedes it. At the same time the throwing motion begins, a terrific push is given with the right leg as the hips, trunk, and shoulders rotate sharply to the left.

A complete follow-through is important to insure maximum distance and control. As the weight shifts completely to the left leg upon release of the ball, the right leg comes around and the right arm is brought across the front of the body, the thrower finishing with the right hand near the left knee.

The muscles primarily responsible for throwing a ball are the abductors of the shoulder girdle (serratus anterior), the horizontal flexors of the shoulder (anterior deltoid, pectoralis major), the inward rotators of the shoulder (subscapularis, teres major), the extensor of the elbow (triceps), the pronators of the forearm (pronator quadratus, pronator teres), and the flexors of the wrist (flexor carpi group). The muscles of the trunk and legs are also very valuable for balance, push-off, and body rotation.

It is obvious that throwing a baseball is not purely a matter of strength. The best arms are those that are able to explode with speed and strength at precisely the right instant, the action resembling that of a buggy-whip. Therefore, the specific throwing muscles should be trained through resistive exercises, but the greater part of the lifting program should be devoted to exercises that require a combined movement of many muscles used in throwing. It is also noted that throwing a baseball is a fine skill and should be practiced accordingly. Additional strength will mean little in throwing if the skill itself is performed improperly. During the weight-training program, practice correct throwing regularly.

SUPPLEMENTARY EXERCISES AND CONDITIONING DRILLS

A large number of drills specifically designed to improve the power, strength, and flexibility involved in baseball skills are available. In training to improve one's ability in baseball, as in other sports, it is advisable to relate the strength and power gained through resistive exercise to the immediate skill for which one is training. Therefore, in training for baseball, a program of conditioning is needed which will develop strength, power, and coordination in the desired skills of hitting, throwing, and running. Here we concentrate on hitting and throwing. Running drills are described in Chapter 10.

Conditioning Drills for Hitting

39. Swinging a weighted bat
A hole is bored in the large end of a broken or chipped bat. An ounce of hot lead is poured into the hole and allowed to dry and solidify. Weight as many as ten bats with this method, adding an additional ounce to each one. Assume a normal batting stance and practice swinging the bat levelly, concentrating on throwing the loaded end of the bat at an imaginary ball.

Beginning with a 32-ounce bat the weight should increase in units so that the heaviest bat is 43 ounces. It is usually inadvisable to weight the bats more heavily. If the bat is too heavily weighted the large muscles of the body begin to assume a disproportionate amount of the swinging load, instead of allowing the overload to strengthen the smaller wrist and forearm muscles.

40. Wrist pronator

Load a dumbbell at one end and grasp it at the other. Allow the arm to rest on a table, the forearm extending straight out. Allow the weight of the bar to carry the forearm to maximum supination (palm facing up). Turn the arm quickly to a pronated position (palm facing down), the weighted end of the dumbbell describing an arc. Repeat with the other wrist.

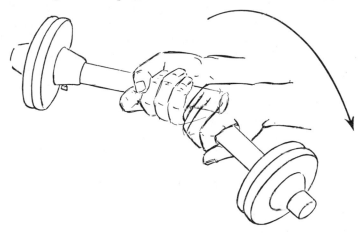

Figure 63. Wrist Pronator

A commercial wrist pronator-supinator is available that attaches to the wall of a gymnasium. An extended handle is turned against resistance, much like a screwdriver. Resistance can be increased by adjusting a screw but the resistance changes are not measurable. The weighted dumbbell is recommended because the overload can gradually be increased by adding to the weights on the end of the dumbbell.

41. Wrist roller

The best way to develop powerful forearms and wrists is to perform wrist rollers using the equipment illustrated in Figure 8. If a large group is training, a faster way is to have two players face each other, one holding a bat, with hands well spread. The other player grasps the bat in the middle and twists it toward himself for six seconds, the first player providing the resistance. Perform two such repetitions, then switch assignments. If the player is training alone, the same exercise can be performed by grasping a parallel bar, or some similar object, instead of a bat.

42. Hip swing

To develop the hip rotation essential to powerful hitting the hip swing drill with resistance is suggested. Place the barbell across the lower back and hold it in that position with the arms, the barbell lying in the crook of the elbow joints. Assume a normal batting stance and rotate to one side. Swing the hips and trunk as you would in hitting a ball, using the muscles of the hips and trunk only. Reverse the action and swing back to the original position.

Skill Drills for Hitting

43. Bat swing

Hold the bat correctly and assume a normal batting stance. Swing at an imaginary ball, attempting to drive the bat through the ball about a foot out in front of the body. The weight should drive against the front leg as the bat meets the imaginary ball. Vary the height of the imaginary ball so that a level swing may be practiced at all heights between the knees and the armpits. A large mirror can also be used by the player to check his form.

44. Wrist break

Drill a ½-inch hole through the center of a ball and through a point one inch from the hitting end of a bat. Loop a heavy wire through the bat and ball and solder it together. The ball should be no closer than 5 inches from the end of the bat.

Place the ball behind the bat and assume a normal batting stance. Swing the bat as if hitting the ball, causing the attached ball to loop around the front of the bat. Concentrate on the wrist snap so that the ball actually hits on the front of the bat.

45. Batting tee

Hang a net or canvas so that a ball may be hit into it without bouncing off. Paint a home plate on the floor about 6 feet away and place a batting tee on the front edge. Place a ball on the tee and take a proper batting stance. Drive the ball off the tee into the net using a normal swing.

Conditioning Drills for Throwing

46. Throwing weighted ball

Bore a small hole halfway through an old baseball and pour an ounce of hot lead into it, allowing it to solidify before using. Weight as many as ten balls with this method, adding an additional ounce to each one. The heaviest ball should contain ten ounces of lead.

Throw the lightest ball easily at first, then, very gradually, throw it harder and harder until it is being thrown as hard as possible with no soreness. This may take one to several weeks. Graduate to the next heaviest ball and proceed in the same manner, catching with a teammate at a distance of 60 feet. Concentrate on throwing the ball properly, getting a full wrist snap into each throw.

47. Wall pulley

Face away from the wall pulleys and grasp a handle in each hand, holding them in a throwing position behind the head. Using a throwing motion, alternately extend the arms the desired number of repetitions. Isokinetic equipment is now available that attaches to the wall and operates on the same principle as the wall pulley, except the resistance is much more uniform. This equipment is highly recommended.

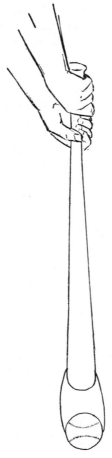

Figure 64. Wrist Break

Skill Drills for Throwing

48.   Play catch

Two players stand 40 feet apart and toss the ball back and forth. As their arms become conditioned they should move back to 60 feet. As they throw to each other they should always practice throwing form and accuracy. The latter can be improved by throwing to a target, such as the partner's left knee, his right foot, his cap, etc. Outfielders and infielders should gradually move back to 120 feet for their throwing sessions.

General Conditioning Drills

49. Wind sprint

The player takes a starting position similar to that taken in stealing a base. Starting with a crossover step, he sprints 30 yards, slowing down gradually and walking 30 yards. The drill should concentrate on a quick start followed by a short burst of speed.

50. Ball pass

Two players stand 30 yards apart; one takes a fielding position and, starting with a crossover step, runs laterally across the field as if chasing a batted ball. The other player throws him the ball, far enough ahead of him so that he must run as fast as possible to catch it. The players then reverse assignments and work their way down the field in this manner. Practice sprinting on the toes, using good running form, and not reaching out to catch the ball until the last stride.

51. Dumbbell circle

For increased flexibility, arm-circling exercises using lightly loaded dumbbells are recommended. Grasping each at its end, hold a dumbbell in each hand. Exercise the shoulders first by performing full arm circles, forward and backward. Then perform the same exercise at the wrist joints. Five circles in each direction at each joint are usually enough.

General Skill Drills

52. Bunting bat control

This drill helps train players to see the ball to the bat, and to train the hand–eye coordination necessary for good bunting. Two players face each other about 5 feet apart, each holding a bat with a grip similar to that used in bunting. A ball is tossed to one of the players who in turn bunts it across to the other. He bunts it back and they attempt to keep the ball in the air by bunting it back and forth.

53. Ball pick-up

This is one of the very best baseball conditioning drills, providing good practice in lateral movement and fielding. Two players take a crouch position facing each other, one holding a ball in each hand. He rolls a ball to one side of his partner, who catches it and tosses it back. As the first ball is being returned he rolls a second ball to the opposite side and the retriever follows the same procedure. Continue rolling the balls, the partner returning them. Start with one set of twenty-five pick-ups and gradually increase.

54. Pepper game

This is an excellent drill for practicing hitting and fielding and for conditioning the body. Have one player (never more than two) face the batter about 5 yards away. He throws a ball to the batter, who hits it back. The batter concentrates on watching the ball meet the bat squarely and controlling the direction of his hit. The thrower concentrates on fielding the ball and regaining his throwing position in a smooth but rapid manner.

55. Conditioning games

Handball is the very best conditioning game for baseball. Every movement performed in baseball is also performed in handball. A fast game of singles helps to develop hand-eye coordination, agility, footwork, and general body condition. It should be played at least three or four times a week during the off-season training period. Many major league players maintain good condition by playing during the off-season. The stiffer the competition, the greater the benefits.

If handball courts are not available, basketball is an acceptable substitute, although it doesn't simulate baseball skills nearly so closely as handball.

OFF-SEASON PROGRAM

In order to obtain the most desirable results, an off-season weight-training program should be conducted for at least three months. This length of time enables the player to make truly significant gains in strength and power. The first month is devoted primarily to a basic training program supplemented by baseball drills. The scope and the intensity of the program are increased during the second and third months by expanding the number of exercises, concentrating especially on the arms and shoulders.

The programs outlined are basically those we have used. If they are employed they should be followed in the order listed. If the conditions or equipment are not suitable to conduct such a program, other exercises may be inserted. Some good ones to use as replacements, or as mere "routine breakers," are the Dead Lift, Straight Legs (25), Straight Arm Pullover (23), Tricep (17), Wall Pulley (47), and the Shoulder Dip (19).

The program is the same for pitchers, catchers, infielders, and outfielders. There is, however, a difference for the overweight and underweight players. The underweight players should further restrict the alternate day program while the overweight players should engage in a more intensive one, with special emphasis on handball, running, and sit-ups.

Lifting Program, First Two Weeks

Exercise	Repetitions	Sets
Warm-up		
1. Jogging	1 lap	1
2. Ball pick-up (53)	25	1
3. Dumbbell circle (51)	5 each position	1
4. Hip swing (42)	10	1

5. Wrist roller (41)	2	1
Power Exercises		
1. Modified clean & power press (2, 4)	10	1
2. Power curl (3)	10	1
3. Squat jump (1)	10	1
4. Dumbbell swing (5)	10	1
Basic Exercises		
1. Squat (28)	15-15	2
2. Bench press (22)	10-10	2
3. Sit-up (26)	25-25	2
4. Overhead press (11)	10-10	2
5. Two-arm curl (16)	10-10	2
6. Lateral raise, supine (24)	10-10	2
7. Straight-arm pullover (23)	10-10	2

Lifting Program, After First Two Weeks

Exercise	*Repetitions*	*Sets*
Warm-up		
1. Jogging	1 lap	1
2. Ball pick-up (53)	25	1
3. Dumbbell circle (51)	5 each position	1
4. Hip swing (42)	10	1
5. Wrist roller (41)	2	1
Power Exercises		
1. Modified clean & power press (2, 4)	10	1
2. Power curl (3)	10	1
3. Squat jump (1)	15	1
4. Dumbbell swing (5)	10	1
Basic Exercises		
1. Squat (28)	15-maximum	2
2. Bench press (22)	10-maximum	2
3. Dead lift, straight legs (25)	15-15	2
4. Sit-up (26)	25-maximum to 100	2
5. Overhead press (11)	10-maximum	2
6. Two-arm curl (16)	10-maximum	2
7. Lateral raise, supine (24)	10-10	2
8. Wrist pronator (40)	10-10	2
9. Wrist curl (20)	10-maximum	2

Alternate-day Program

If weight-training exercises are practiced exclusively there exists a possibility that the movement patterns learned in weight training may override those previously learned in baseball and possibly interfere with them. To prevent this a brief alternate-day program of baseball drills, such as outlined below, should be practiced. This program should be followed by the outlined program of functional isometrics on the power rack at least two days a week.

Exercise	Repetitions	Sets
1. Jogging	1 lap	1
2. Ball pick-up (53)	25	1
3. Play catch (48)	5 minutes	1
4. Bat swing (43)	15	2
5. Wind sprint (49)	5	1
6. Handball (or basketball) (55)	Two games, singles	

Power Rack Program (Hold each exercise approximately seven seconds)
1. Heel-raise (38)
2. Overhead press (34)
3. Curl (33)
4. Upright rowing (35)
5. Bench press (37)
6. Dead lift (36)

PRE-SEASON PROGRAM

This program is designed to have the players ready to go at top speed on the first outdoor practice day. In high school and college seasons this is extremely important. It should be noted that the program is not intended to go beyond the first outdoor practice period. The multitude of offensive and defensive drills, which must be done outdoors, will and should use up the greater part of the time immediately before the season begins. It is assumed that the players have *not* been participating in an off-season program. If they have been following the off-season program they should continue the lifting part of that program for the first three weeks of the pre-season program and should adjust their alternate day program to coincide with the pre-season program.

The first three weeks of the pre-season program of conditioning should be devoted to a wide range of weight-training exercises plus baseball skill and conditioning drills. As the players round into condition the number of weight training exercises is decreased and practice of the baseball skills (hitting, running, throwing, and fielding) is increased. The running should be done outdoors whenever possible to properly condition the legs to the soft ground.

No attempt has been made in this program to differentiate between pitchers and other players. Quite obviously the pitchers should spend more time than is indicated in throwing and running and probably less time in practicing the hitting drills. Their arms should be in condition to throw batting practice without difficulty after the pre-season conditioning program.

Training Program, First Two Weeks

Lifting program

Exercise	Repetitions	Sets
Warm-up		
1. Jogging	1 lap	1
2. Ball pick-up (53)	25	1
3. Dumbbell circle (51)	5 each position	1
4. Hip swing (42)	10	1
5. Wrist roller (41)	2	1
Power Exercises		
1. Modified clean & power press (2, 4)	10	1
2. Power curl (3)	10	1
3. Squat jump (1)	10	1
4. Dumbbell swing (5)	10	1

Basic Exercises

Exercise	Repetitions	Sets
1. Squat (28)	15-15	2
2. Bench press (22)	10-10	2
3. Sit-up (26)	25-25	2
4. Overhead press (11)	10-10	2
5. Two-arm curl (16)	10-10	2
6. Straight-arm pullover (23)	10-10	2
7. Tricep (17)	10-10	2

Alternate-day program

1. Jogging	1 lap	1
2. Ball pick-up (53)	25	1
3. Throwing weighted ball (46)	5-6 minutes	1
4. Wrist break (44)	15	1
5. Bat swing (43)	15	1

6. Wind sprint (49)	5	1
7. Handball (or basketball) (55)	Best of three, singles	1

Training Program, Last Four Weeks

Lifting program

Warm-up

1. Jogging	1 lap	1
2. Ball pick-up (53)	25	1
3. Dumbbell circle (51)	5 each position	1
4. Hip swing (42)	10	1
5. Play catch (48)	10-12 minutes	1
6. Wrist roller (41)	3	1

Power Exercises

1. Power curl (3)	10	1
2. Power press (4)	10	1
3. Dumbbell swing (5)	10	1

Basic Exercises

Exercise	Repetitions	Sets
1. Modified clean (2)	10	1
2. Squat (28)	15-15	2
3. Sit-up (26)	25-25	2
4. Two-arm curl (16)	10-10	2
5. Bench press (22)	10-10	2
6. Straight-arm pullover (23)	10-10	2
7. Overhead press (11)	10-10	2

Ninth-Inning Drill

1. Ball pick-up (53)	25	2
2. Wind sprint (49)	5, add one each day	1
3. Jogging	1 lap	

Alternate-day program

Exercise	Repetitions	Sets
1. Jogging	1 lap	1
2. Ball pick-up (53)	25	2
3. Play catch (48)	10 minutes	1
4. Bat swing (43)	15	1
5. Pepper game (54)	10 minutes	1
6. Wind sprint (49)	5, add one each day	1
7. Handball (or basketball) (55)	1 game	1

IN-SEASON PROGRAM

As a rule, no attempt is made to conduct a weight-training program during the playing season, because the physical strain of participating in two athletic programs simultaneously is too demanding. However, baseball is unique in this respect. During a season baseball players do not get the physical exercise needed to maintain the physical development they will acquire from a weight-training program. The game simply doesn't provide the opportunity to maintain the strength and power demanded of them at infrequent intervals during the season. Therefore, some method should be provided to maintain the gains derived from the weight-training program without bringing on undue fatigue in the players.

No attempt should be made during the in-season program to increase strength through weight training by adding to the weight in the various exercises. A moderate lifting program, with the aim of maintaining the level of muscular efficiency previously developed through the conditioning program, is more practical. Some experts have established that this can be done by conducting a shortened program on only one – or possibly two – days a week. It is recommended that the in-season program be used only twice a week at the conclusion of the practice sessions. The more desirable days are those that do not precede a playing day, though this is not absolutely necessary. Arrange the exercise days so that at least two days separate them.

It is worthy of mention that catchers should give special emphasis to leg-stretching exercises. Maintaining the squatting position behind the plate over long periods of time will eventually cause the hamstring muscles behind the legs to tighten up, possibly impairing the catchers' running speed. The Dead Lift, Straight Legs (25) is recommended.

Training Program

Exercise	Repetitions	Sets
Power Exercises		
1. Power curl (3)	10	1
2. Squat jump (1)	10	1
3. Power press (4)	10	1
4. Dumbbell swing (5)	10	1
Basic Exercises		
1. Modified clean (2)	10	1
2. Squat (28)	15	1
3. Dead lift, straight legs (25)	10	1
4. Bench press (22)	10	1
5. Sit-up (26)	25	1

6. Overhead press (11)	10	1
7. Two-arm curl (16)	10	1
8. Straight-arm pullover (23)	10	1

THE PROFESSIONAL PLAYER

The off-season and pre-season training programs previously described in this chapter are applicable to professional players as well as those in high school and college. There is a big difference, however, in their playing schedules. The high school and college teams usually play only two or three times a week and for little more than eight weeks. It is a relatively simple matter for them to conduct an in-season weight-training program. The professional player, on the other hand, plays almost every day for more than six months. It is very difficult for the professional to find time for weight training.

A program of power exercises is recommended for the professional during the season because it trains the explosive muscular contraction so vital to baseball success. No attempt should be made to increase the amount of weight on the bar and no more than the recommended number of exercises is advisable. The player should train twice a week, one of the sessions coming on an off day if possible. If there are no off days, the training should be at around 9:00 A.M. on the day of a night game. The Wrist Rollers (41) are practiced every day by some players with excellent results. If the forearms and wrists are weak, this exercise certainly should be done each day.

Training Program

Exercise	Repetitions	Sets
1. Modified clean (2)	10	1
2. Power press (4)	10	1
3. Sit-up (26)	25	1
4. Power curl (3)	10	1
5. Dumbbell swing (5)	10	1
6. Wrist rollers (41)	2	1
7. Two-arm curl (16)	10	1
8. Overhead press (11)	10	1

THE SORE ARM IN BASEBALL

The first year a weight-training program was attempted with Wake Forest baseball players only the pitchers and catchers were asked to participate. The program was similar to the pre-season one outlined in this chapter. Its aim was to so condition the pitchers during a concentrated six-week period that they could take a turn pitching batting practice on the first day of the regular outdoor practice. The three objectives of the program were: (1) to keep the joints loose through stretching exercises so that the whiplike action necessary for good pitching would be maintained; (2) to develop general body strength and muscle tonus through the basic strength and power exercises; and (3) to give specific attention, through additional exercises, to the muscle groups that receive a concentrated stress during the throwing movement.

The results of the program were gratifying. Not a single pitcher or catcher had arm trouble that spring. The infielders and outfielders who had used the more conventional-type program of running, throwing, and light exercises were not quite so fortunate. Admittedly, there is nothing scientific about these results. It could have happened by chance. We were convinced, however, to the extent that the entire squad was put on the same program the following spring, with excellent results.

One should not interpret the previous example as meaning that weight training will prevent sore arms in baseball. It will do so only if it is part of a sound program of conditioning which includes instruction on proper warm-up, proper dress, cooling off, etc. Weight training conditions the muscles to perform under adverse conditions, but it should be used in conjunction with other phases of the training program — not as a substitute for them.

If a player has a sore arm he should usually be examined by an orthopedist, who should suggest any subsequent treatment necessary. If exercise is recommended, the amount and intensity will probably be prescribed. If not, be sure to start with low resistance and build up gradually. Boys often develop sore arms during the cooler nights of August and September and the entire winter can be devoted to rehabilitation. We have had good success using the off-season training program suggested in this chapter.

Stretching exercises are sometimes a helpful supplement for arm conditioning. The best way to stretch and relax the arm muscles is to grasp an overhead bar and hang from it, bearing only part of the weight with the feet. This type of exercise is usually used during the season to relieve tightness in the shoulder.

SELECTED REFERENCES

Allen, Archie P., *Handbook of Baseball Drills.* Englewood Cliffs, N.J.: Prentice-Hall, Inc., 1959.

Alston, Walter, and Don Weiskopf, *The Complete Baseball Handbook.* Boston: Allyn and Bacon, Inc., 1972.

DeLorme, Thomas L., and Arthur L. Watkins, *Progressive Resistive Exercise.* New York: Appleton-Century-Crofts, Inc., 1951.

Hawley, Gertrude, *An Anatomical Analysis of Sports.* New York: A. S. Barnes and Company, 1940.

Larson, Leonard A., *Encyclopedia of Sport Sciences and Medicine.* New York: The Macmillan Company, 1971.

Morehouse, Laurence E., and Philip J. Rasch, *Scientific Basis of Athletic Training.* Philadelphia: W. B. Saunders Company, 1958.

Wells, Katherine F., *Kinesiology,* 3rd ed. Philadelphia: W. B. Saunders Company, 1960.

7

WEIGHT TRAINING
IN BASKETBALL

Many qualities go into the making of a good basketball player. Agility, intelligence, reaction, coordination and desire are some of the more important. The truth is that these qualities amount to very little if the player isn't properly conditioned. He must train to such a fine point that he can play a full game at top speed and not be too exhausted. Such training requires a great deal of running to develop stamina and muscular endurance. A relatively strong player can play his way into top condition in a few weeks, but many of the weaker boys will never achieve the endurance and stamina they need because they lack the muscular strength that is the foundation of good conditioning.

Many very skilled basketball players are not strong enough to be successful. It's true that a basketball is relatively light, and to shoot, pass, or dribble it does not require much strength. However, the situation is far different when opposition is provided. The player must control the ball while being guarded closely by an opponent; he must make goals in spite of slapping hands; he must stand his ground under the basket and jump high to retrieve a rebound; and to be successful he must protect the ball from aggressive opposition. Superior strength will not accomplish these things for a player if he lacks desire, aggressiveness, coordination, agility, or any of the other characteristics important to basketball success. It is a fact, however, that the best basketball players in the game today, excluding only a few of the back court wizards, are strong and powerful athletes.

If a player doesn't have good size and strength, the best way to achieve them is through a well-planned weight-training program. Some basketball coaches and players oppose weight training because they feel that being a good shot requires such a fine degree of coordination and "touch" that an increase in strength might be detrimental. Such logic is puzzling. Numerous experiments have been conducted along these lines, and in instances where sensible weight-training programs were conducted the improved strength had no effect on shooting accuracy; in fact, it resulted in improved jumping and rebounding.

Basketball's great Wilt Chamberlain is the best example of the value of strength in basketball. According to Bill Neider, an avid weight trainer who won the gold medal in the shot put at the 1960 Rome Olympics, he has never been beaten at arm wrestling and has only been tied by one man. That man was Wilt Chamberlain.[1] Chamberlain's height and powerful physique give him a tremendous advantage in under-the-board play. Although he may never have weight trained, he has somehow acquired astounding strength to accompany his tremendous size. He can simply overpower the opposition.

Most coaches recognize the need for general body strength in a basketball player. Because the game itself is not designed to develop strength, and yet requires it for success, many have used weights. It has been proven that players usually improve their jumping height three inches — and some as much as six inches — through weight training. Many players at Wake Forest have used a general weight-training program during the off-season, and the Wake Forest coaches have encouraged weight training for many high school players who need additional strength and size. More and more high schools and colleges are following their lead.

DISCUSSION OF SKILLS

Those skills which are fundamental to success in basketball are dribbling, faking, pivoting, guarding, passing, shooting, and rebounding. There are occasions when a specialist in one of the skills can be used to advantage, but this isn't nearly as popular as in football or baseball. Even though a player may re-enter the game as often as he likes, he must remain there as long as the clock continues to run. During this time he will be exposed to a great number of different play situations. Therefore, he must be skilled in all fundamentals of the game if he is going to pull his share of the load.

Basic body strength is necessary to basketball success, though some of the skills, such as dribbling, faking, pivoting, passing, and guarding require only an average amount of strength. Weight training will probably influence these skills only insofar as the player can improve his ability to handle his body weight. The additional strength would improve his muscular endurance. Other skills such as shooting and rebounding can be more noticeably improved through weight training, and are therefore discussed in more detail.

[1] Tex Maule, "The Shotput Explosion," *Sports Illustrated* (April 25, 1960), p. 30.

Shooting

Shooting is unquestionably the most important basketball fundamental. The best ball handlers are relatively unimportant to a team if they aren't able to put the ball in the basket consistently. It takes a great deal of individual and team strategy to clear a player for a shot; when a player gets the opportunity he should therefore be able to score.

What makes a good scorer? Two of the most important aspects are the jumping ability of the shooter and his shooting accuracy. If a player can jump higher than his opponents he has a distinct advantage in shooting because he is closer to the basket and because he has less difficulty in getting the shot off without having it blocked. However, there are many players who shoot well yet don't score well. A player usually must work under very difficult conditions to get a shot at the basket. Especially in the close-in shots the ball, the arms, or the hand are often hit by a guard as the shot is being taken. The stronger, more powerful players nevertheless often make the shot good. Therefore, the best scorers in basketball not only can jump high and shoot accurately, but have the weight to maintain a good court position and the strength to put the ball in the basket even when fouled.

There have been two exceptionally strong men at Wake Forest in the last twenty years: Dick Hemric and Len Chappell. Hemric was the school's first All-American basketball player in 1955. That year he was 6 feet, 6 inches tall and weighed 220 pounds. He wasn't the tallest player ever to play at Wake Forest by any means, but he was one of the strongest. Hemric used his tremendous strength to break every conference scoring record and to set a national record of total points scored by an individual during a four-year career.

The school's next All-American was Len Chappell. As a senior, Chappell was 6 feet, 8 inches tall and weighed 240 pounds, and was equally as powerful as Hemric. Both players hit exceptional percentages from the floor — in fact, better than fifty percent, which shows that their terrific strength didn't hinder their shooting accuracy. They enjoyed an obvious height advantage, but there have been many college basketball players as tall who didn't make All-American. Many could shoot as well or better, yet didn't score as well. This has been true primarily because only a few of these tall players were big and strong. Some of them were actually frail. As a result they were at a tremendous disadvantage in trying to score from close around the basket. It is no accident that two of the four All-Americans in the last twenty years Wake Forest has played the sport have been their biggest and strongest players.

The most satisfying part of the game is shooting, and it is certainly the easiest fundamental to get the players to practice. The two shots used most frequently in the modern game are the one-hand jump shot and the one-hand /-up shot.

1. The jump shot

The jump shot has completely revolutionalized basketball because the change of pace and the quick jump make the shot extremely difficult to guard against. Also, many players have learned to hit an exceptionally high percentage of this type of shot. It is started from a semi-crouch position, the trunk, hips, and knees partly flexed. The ball is held in front of the body with both hands at approximately a chest-high position. The body weight should be well balanced on the balls of the feet with the right foot slightly forward if the shot is being taken with the right hand. The jump is straight up, and the ball is carried to the shooting position by extending the arms over the head. The left hand is to the side of and slightly under the ball, while the shooting hand is behind and under. The elbows are slightly bent. The ball is shot at the peak of the jump by flexing the wrist and fingers and slightly extending the arms at the elbow. The follow-through is effected by allowing the right hand to come forward naturally so that the palm faces the floor.

2. The one-hand lay-up

The one-hand lay-up is the simplest shot in the game if the player isn't being guarded. During a game, however, it is often missed, not only because the fundamentals of the shot haven't been mastered, but quite often because the shot is rushed by the shooter for fear of being hit while in the air. The drive for the basket is started after a dribble or a pass. The player leaves the floor with the left foot last for a right hand shot, completely extending his body and legs. The ball is carried up to the basket with both hands, but the left hand is released a little above shoulder height and aids the body in protecting the ball. The right hand carries the ball to the highest point of the jump and lays it over the rim or against the backboard above the basket. No extra spin is applied. At the height of the jump the legs, body, and right arm are completely extended while the left elbow and shoulder are flexed for balance and ball protection. On the driving lay-ups, the right hand is under the ball and the speed of the drive provides the necessary momentum for the shot. However, many players place the hand directly behind the ball so that the hand and wrist furnish the final momentum for the shot. This method enables the shooter to control the ball better on lay-up shots that start from close around the basket.

The most common mistake in shooting the lay-up is in the jump. It should be a high jump, not a broad jump; a great amount of emphasis should therefore be placed on planting the jumping foot hard on the floor and jumping as high as possible. If possible, gather for the jump by controlling the running speed immediately before the jump.

There are many variations of shots that could be described in detail, but as far as fundamentals and strength are concerned they are very similar to the two described. Most of them are executed by springing from the floor and are attempted under playing conditions that make body weight and arm and shoulder strength very important. The most vital jumping muscles are the hip extensors (gluteus maximus), knee extensors (quadriceps femoris), and the ankle plantar flexors (gastrocnemius, soleus).

Much has been said about the need for strength in the arms and shoulders to maintain control of the ball. No specific muscle groups are indicated in this area, however, because all of the muscles must be well-developed in order to steady the arms for accurate shooting. The extensors of the arms and shoulders actually carry the ball high for the shot, but the arm flexors furnish the force to bring down a rebound and control it afterwards. General muscular development in the arms and shoulders is therefore necessary.

Hand strength is of utmost importance. In fact, in no other sport is the flexor strength of the hands and wrists (flexor carpi group) so important as it is in basketball. If a player doesn't have strong hands he has very little chance to be a good basketball player. Of course, he must practice long hours to develop his touch and shooting accuracy, but he should spend a proportionate amount of time developing the strength of his hands and wrists.

Rebounding

Probably no axiom holds so true in basketball as "control the backboards and you control the game." Size and height are major assets to rebounding ability, but the good rebounder has other necessary qualifications. He has the courage and aggressiveness to fight the flying elbows and knees under the basket, catlike reaction and agility to scramble to a key position, a fine degree of coordination to time the jump perfectly, powerful leg spring to jump high enough for the rebound, and powerful arms and hands to maintain possession and control of the ball.

There are three main divisions in rebounding technique: position, jump, and ball control. Good position is basic to good rebounding. A good rebounder won't allow an opponent to push him too far under the basket, nor will he allow himself to be blocked out too far from the basket. His best position is one between his opponent and the basket, and, if he is able to get it, he holds his ground.

In preparing to jump for the ball, the body should be crouched with the weight on the balls of the feet. In this ready position the head and chin should be up, the shoulders retracted, the arms slightly abducted, the hips and knees well flexed, the hips down, and the feet slightly apart. Such a position assures a good base for position and spring.

The jump is made with a powerful extension of the hips, knees, and ankles, and by throwing the arms up as high as possible. Though most jumping for a rebound is done from a standing-still position, more height can be attained when several steps are taken before the jump. This allows the jumper to plant his feet hard on the floor, readying the leg muscles for a maximum spring. The steps before the jump should be short ones without too much forward speed, so that all of the spring can be exploded upward. It is usually necessary to be able to control the body during the jump so the rebounder can clear the area without fouling.

Under the defensive backboard the player should grab the ball with two hands, usually coming down with the legs spread and the body flexed at the waist in a jackknifed position, shielding the ball from the opponent. It should be cleared from the congested area as soon as possible with a pass out or a dribble. If, under the offensive board there is no chance to grab the rebound, he should attempt to tip the ball in. An inch or two of added height can be attained by tipping the ball with one hand, controlling the ball on the fingertips and shooting with a flick of the wrists and fingers.

Though leg spring is probably the most desirable physical asset for rebounding, the good rebounder must be big and strong to hold his ground before the jump, and the jump itself must be a coordinated movement of the entire body — not just an uncoiling of the legs. The key muscles in jumping are the knee extensors (quadriceps femoris), ankle extensors (gastrocnemius, soleus), and the extensors of the hip (gluteus maximus). The flexors of the great toes (flexor hallucis longus) provide the final "push-off" in the jump. The arms drive up hard and the lower back extends forcefully to assist in the jump, emphasizing the need for a full body movement.

The amount of crouch and consequently the amount of spring a player can get is proportional to the strength of the extensor muscles of the knee and ankle.[2] In other words, in jumping for a rebound, the stronger the muscles the greater can be the crouch for the most height in the jump. This means that basketball players should spend extra time, especially during the off-season, to strengthen the quadriceps and the calf muscles so that they can add to their jumping ability. Not only will they be able to jump higher on the first jump, but they will be able to get up higher and more quickly on the second and third efforts. Often, the rebound is not controlled until the second or third jump, and the player with the stronger legs will get the job done.

SUPPLEMENTARY EXERCISES AND DRILLS

Although entire books have been written on basketball drills, only a small core of individual drills for shooting, rebounding, and conditioning is necessary if a player will practice them faithfully during the off-season. Many people contend that good shooters are born, not made. However, the very fact that shooting percentages have increased tremendously in the past twenty years and continue to go up each year attests to the fact that shooting accuracy can be learned. Certainly there are many "naturals," but a lot of practice is needed to hit a good percentage of shots. The outstanding players today play almost the entire year round.

Many conferences restrict fall and spring basketball on an organized basis because it interferes with other sports. However, many players do not participate

---

[2]John W. Bunn, *Scientific Principles of Coaching,* Englewood Cliffs, N.J.: Prent' Hall, Inc. (1955), p. 90.

in other sports and wish to reach their full potential in basketball. Two or three games a week leave comparatively little time for work on fundamentals during a season because much of the practice periods must be spent on team offense and defense.

The drills presented in this chapter are individual-type drills for practice by only one, two, or several players. They should be practiced on the days the players don't weight train so that the arm and leg strength derived from the training program can be applied to their basketball skills. Special drills for jump shooting, lay-up shooting, and rebounding are offered because increased strength will directly influence these skills if they are practiced correctly. Some conditioning drills are included which can be used during the pre-season training program.

Drills for Shooting

56. Lay-up drills

One of the most important fundamentals in shooting the lay-up is jumping as high as possible. Many players broad jump and flip the ball at the basket as they go by. A good way to break the broad jump habit is to place an obstacle (chair) underneath the backboard. The player should drive straight for the chair, jump high for the lay-up, and come down in front of the chair without touching it. Vary the angle and speed of the drive, placing the chair further beneath the basket for faster drives. For the drive down the middle, place another chair in front of the basket and force the shooter to one side or the other making him bank the shot.

57. Catch rebound

This is another good drill to force the player to jump high for the lay-up and to control his speed as he goes up for the shot. The player should drive hard at the basket, taking a long last stride and planting the takeoff foot hard on the floor before jumping as high as possible. He should come straight down after the shot and try to get the rebound before it hits the floor. Strive to increase the speed of the drive and the height of the jump.

58. Quick stop and jump

One of the most important offensive moves in the modern game is to drive off a screen, stop quickly, and take the jump shot. A player should practice for long hours the drive and jump shot, dribbling to the right for one shot and back to the left for another. A chair (or another player) may be placed in front of the player for use as a screen. He should drive close to the chair, and as he clears it, stop quickly and take the jump shot. Vary the drill by having the player drive straight at the chair and stop and jump. This practice will force him to make his jump up instead of out, thus getting higher off the floor for the shot. It should also prevent his falling into his man after the shot. If players can work in pairs they should screen for each other instead of using the chairs. The best way to do this is to have one pass to the other and move toward him, getting a return pass as he approaches, drives by, and takes the jump shot.

59.   Twenty-one

This is a competitive drill in which a variety of shots may be used. It is particularly valuable for practicing the jump shot. Give a ball to each player and have him shoot from a designated distance (no further than the top of the keyhole). The first player to hit twenty-one shots first wins. The game may be varied by having each player shoot a long jump shot and follow it, shooting a short jump shot from the place where he retrieves the ball. The long shot counts two points; the short shot counts one point. Another variation is making the short shot a lay-up, delaying the scoring until the jump shot has been made. If only one ball is available, the players can use the same ball, alternating turns.

Drills for Rebounding

60.   Rebound machine

The rebound machine is excellent for determining the highest jumpers on the team and for training a player in the proper form for rebounding. The

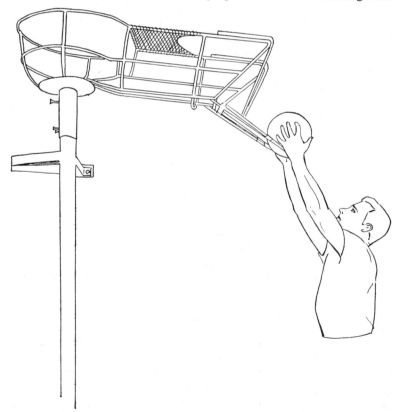

Figure 65. Rebound Machine

machine should at first be set at an attainable height, and the player should try twenty jumps each day, ten from a standing position and ten using a two- or three-step start. He should jackknife as he comes down with the ball and pivot and dribble or pass out when he hits the floor. A record of the jumps should be made and compared from day to day. The machine should gradually be raised until the player is jumping for his best height each time.

If a rebound machine is not available, a useful drill is the vertical jump. Place a blackboard against the wall extending upward from the six-foot mark. The player stands flat-footed against the wall and reaches as high as possible, making a chalk mark at that point. He then backs off and jumps as high as possible, making another mark at the new point. The difference between the two marks is then measured. Practice the jumps as suggested for the rebound machine. Strive for improvement but don't be too impressed by the distance of the jump; the actual height of the jump is more indicative of the jumper's value as a rebounder. Measure all jumps, because knowledge of the height of the last jump can be valuable in judging leg strength, endurance, and general condition.

61. Tipping endurance

To develop leg endurance and fingertip control, this drill should be practiced each day. One, two, or three players should line up in front of the goal. The first man in line tosses the ball against the backboard and taps it against the board five times, jumping high each time. On the sixth jump the next man takes a turn before they rotate again. The number of repetitions should be increased by one each day until a player is able to do at least twenty-five good tips in succession.

62. Tipping ring

This is an excellent drill for developing the timing of the jump. A small inner ring measuring 16 inches across the inside is attached so that the inner ring is slightly higher than the outer. A player is placed on one, two, or three sides and the ball is tossed up on the boards. Each man attempts to tip the ball in the goal as it comes to his area of the basket. The players should rotate periodically.

Some teams use a tipping cover instead of the ring. The cover is secured tightly over the goal so the ball cannot go through and the drill is performed as with the tipping ring.

General Conditioning Drills

63. Rope skip

Although rope-skipping is discussed in other chapters, it is worthy of special mention in basketball. Because it develops the calves of the legs, the rope skip is an extremely valuable exercise for agility and leg spring. Nothing fancy is necessary, just jumping on the balls of the feet at different speeds. During the early stages of the program, players should skip for three to four minutes daily. Later they may drop to two minutes, and some may stop after the season begins; but the big men should continue practicing throughout most of the season.

Ropes should be checked out to these men so they can practice as often as possible.

64. Medicine ball

The medicine ball is often used to practice passing fundamentals and to build strength. There is some doubt as to its value in strength-building, but it has some value as a routine breaker, and because it can't be dribbled it is very effective for use in a passing drill. The six-pound medicine ball is merely substituted for the basketball in the passing drills during the early conditioning program. It should not be used immediately before or during the season. A very enjoyable drill is to alternate the medicine ball and a basketball. The players enjoy their temporary feeling of strength in passing the basketball.

65. Maze run

An excellent way of motivating the players to run and to increase agility is having them practice the maze run. Six chairs are placed on the floor as illustrated. The player sprints through the course as rapidly as possible. This drill may be varied in any number of ways. One is to require the player to come back through the maze to the starting line, or have him dribble through the course. Another very good variation is to have the player run through the maze backwards. He should use good defensive footwork, constantly feeling for the chairs behind him and using peripheral vision to see the chairs without turning his head. All aspects of this drill should be performed against the stop watch periodically to encourage improvement.

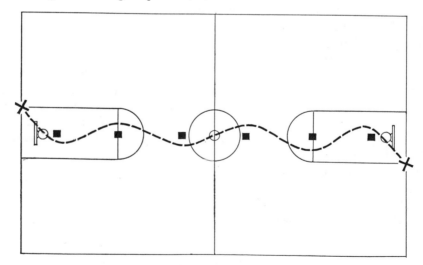

Figure 66. Maze Run

66. Endurance drill

This drill is one of the few that develops agility and endurance, and is very good during the pre-season conditioning program. The player starts at the end of the court and sprints to the foul line. After touching it he returns to the end line. Then he sprints to the middle of the court and back; then to the other foul line and back; then to the other end line and back. The players should not run in circles when they change directions, but should hit hard on one foot and drive back in the opposite direction. Time the players to determine which can go through fastest and to see if they are improving. When they are in top shape they should be able to go through the drill at top speed. A good modification of the drill is to have the players dribble through, changing hands as they change directions.

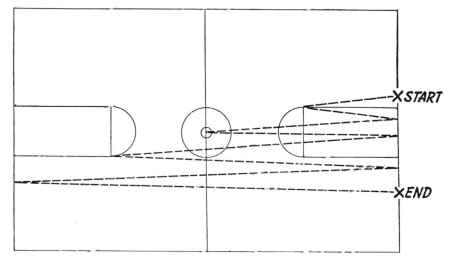

Figure 67. Endurance Drill

General Skill Drills

67. One on one

This is an excellent drill to practice individual offensive and defensive fundamentals and is the very best competitive basketball drill. One player takes the ball at the top of the keyhole and attempts to score by faking, driving, etc., against an opponent. As long as he scores he gets to keep the ball and try again. If he misses he tries to follow the shot. If the opponent gets the rebound he must take the ball behind the free throw line before attempting a shot. The player who scores ten baskets first is the winner.

OFF-SEASON PROGRAM

The off-season weight-training program for basketball can be done in the spring or summer. The primary considerations should be the amount of uninterrupted time available and the mental attitude of the players. If the program is planned for the spring it is a good idea for the players to take a week or ten days off at the completion of the season to relax physically and mentally. Those who plan to follow the program on an individual basis will probably find more free time in the summer. For best results the program should last about three months.

The program presented is one that many of our boys have used at Wake Forest. It is almost impossible to outline a general program that meets the demands of all squads with all types of body builds and with different facilities. However, this program should be acceptable for most situations in the first month. During this period the muscles are conditioned, the lifts and the routine are learned, and training habits are formed. During the second and third months other exercises may be inserted according to the individual weaknesses of the players, or simply as substitute exercises for variety. After the first three weeks the weight loads should be increased according to the 10-maximum program.

The program is the same for forwards, guards, and centers. However, there is a big difference between overweight and underweight players. Much has been said about the ability of an individual to gain strength through weight training, but almost as important in basketball is the fact that regular lifting will also help one gain weight if good diet and regular hours are maintained. This is especially important in shooting and rebounding, and the thinner players should make every effort to fill out and strengthen their bodies. The underweight player should not hesitate in varying the program to better accomplish this. The Bench Press (22) exercise should be performed an extra set, and three sets of Dead Lifts (29), and two sets of Lateral Raises, Supine (24) are also needed. The Dead Lift, Streight Legs can be eliminated and the alternate-day program should be made less intensive.

The overweight player should do extra sets of Squat Jumps (1), Sit-Ups without weight (26), and Vertical Jumps (61). He will also need to participate in a vigorous alternate-day program of general skill and conditioning drills and a power rack program of functional isometrics. Basketball players who aren't strong should work with weights until they have acquired the necessary strength and power to be good players. By the same token there are a few boys who have superior strength and lack the fundamental skill to be good players. They should spend the majority of their off-season time participating in agility and conditioning drills and practicing basketball skills — not in lifting weights. If they want to lift they should practice a general conditioning program to maintain their strength and keep the muscles in proper tone.

Lifting Program

Exercise	Repetitions	Sets
Warm-up		
1. Jogging	1 lap	1
2. Alternate toe touches	10	1
3. Arm circling	5 each way	1

4. Trunk rotation	5 each way	1
5. Squat thrust	10	1

Power Exercises

1. Squat jump (1)	15	1
2. Sit-up (with wt.) (26)	25	1
3. Tipping endurance (61)	20 (10 each hand)	1

Basic Exercises

1. Squat (28)	15-maximum	2
2. Bench press (22)	10-maximum	2
3. Sit-up (speed) (26)	25-maximum to 100	2
4. Overhead press (11)	10-maximum	2
5. Two-arm curl (16)	10-maximum	2
6. Dead lift, straight legs (25)	15-15	2
7. Rowing upright (13)	10-maximum	2
8. Heel-raise (30)	15-maximum	2
9. Wrist curl (20)	10-maximum	2

Alternate-day Program

Shooting a basketball with accuracy requires a lot of practice, whether a player is weight training or not. Therefore, shooting baskets is one skill a player should practice the year round. Other skills as well should be practiced, but not to the same extent. The player's ability should determine the amount of work he should do on alternate lifting days. The plan outlined below is a minimum program and should be practiced at least twice a week by all of the players in the program. Some will need much more work in certain drills.

Alternate-day program

Exercise	Repetitions	Sets
1. Jogging	1 lap	1
2. Rebound machine (60)	20	1
3. Rope skip (63)	4 minutes	1
4. Maze run (65)	1 forward, 1 backward, 1 forward & return	1
5. Quick stop & jump (58)	7-8 minutes	1
6. Twenty-one (59)	Best of 2 of 3 games	1
7. One on one (67)	Best of 2 of 3 games	1

Power Rack Program (Hold each exercise approximately seven seconds)

1. Heel-raise (38)
2. Overhead press (34)

3. Curl (33)
4. Upright rowing (35)
5. Dead lift (36)

PRE-SEASON PROGRAM

Six weeks before official practice begins is ample time to get a squad in top physical condition. This pre-season program is offered as a guide for the coach to condition his squad so that the official practice sessions can be devoted to the fundamentals of basketball and to team offense and defense. If a training program of this nature is followed, the players will lose little time from sore muscles, blisters, and lack of stamina. Although there might be a tendency to take a few days off before the regular practices begin, this should be discouraged. It takes only a few days to get out of condition again.

During the first three weeks the emphasis is on a general lifting program with a special concentration of exercises on the legs. Some basketball drills are used as a warm-up period. All drills involving shooting, passing, or dribbling should be done *before* the weight-training exercises, because the muscles will be too tired to do such drills immediately after lifting. Some extra running drills are included at the end of the training session to start building the wind. These are referred to on the program as second-half drills.

During the last three weeks the program is broadened to include more running. So that this program can be completed in approximately the same length of time, the lifting exercises are reduced to one set, with the exception of the Heel-Raise (38) and Squat (28). The second-half drills become a very important part of the program during this stage. The Maze Run (65) and Endurance Drill (66) should be run each day, and the number of repetitions should be increased until the player is in top condition. These drills should always be done on the basketball court in order to condition the player's feet and legs to the hard floor.

The alternate-day program follows the same general pattern as on lifting days. During the first three weeks the program consists of a variety of skill and conditioning drills. During the latter stages of the program more time should be devoted to half-court games and endurance drills, adding to the latter as endurance improves.

The conditioning program is hard work and requires a great amount of physical punishment before a player is in shape. Much of the torture can be eliminated from the program if a variety of drills is used, encouraging competition in all phases of the program. Besides the games that are suggested in the program, other competitive games and drills may be used. Cross-country running is a part of many programs. Volleyball is also good. If courts are available, handball is an excellent conditioner because the movements closely resemble those in defensive basketball. Relay races are good, and some coaches also require their players to shadowbox. Others are requiring modern dance, which can be excellent for the awkward player if instruction is good and if the players are properly indoctrinated.

Training Program, First Three Weeks

Lifting program

Exercise	Repetitions	Sets
Warm-up		
1. Jogging	1 lap	1
2. Rebound machine (60)	10	1
3. Rope skip (63)	2 minutes	1
4. Quick stop & jump (58)	5 minutes	1
5. Twenty-one (59)	Best 2 of 3 games	1
Power Exercises		
1. Modified clean (2)	10	1
2. Squat jump (1)	10	1
3. Power curl (3)	10	1
Basic Exercises		
1. Squat (28)	15-maximum	2
2. Sit-up (26)	25-25	2
3. Heel-raise (30)	15-maximum	2
4. Overhead press (11)	10-maximum	2
5. Two-arm curl (16)	10-maximum	2
6. Dead lift, Straight legs (25)	15-15	2
7. Rowing upright (13)	10-maximum	2
Second-Half Drills		
1. Wind sprints (58)	5	1
2. Jogging	Half Mile	1

Alternate-day program

1. Jogging	1 lap	1
2. Rope skip (63)	2 minutes	1
3. Rebound machine (60)	20	1
4. Quick stop & jump (58)	5 minutes	1
5. Tipping ring (62)	5 minutes	1
6. One on one (67)	Best 2 of 3 games	1
7. Half-court game	30 minutes	1

Power Rack Program (Hold each exercise approximately seven seconds)
1. Heel-raise (38)
2. Overhead press (34)
3. Curl (33)
4. Upright rowing (35)
5. Dead lift (36)

Jogging

In the pre-season program it is important to begin working to improve stamina and endurance. During the first three weeks a minimum of two miles should be run as a part of the alternate-day program. It is suggested that this be done by alternately running and jogging 440-yard laps, taking minimum rest periods during the first three-week program.

Training Program, Last Three Weeks

Lifting program

Exercise	*Repetitions*	*Sets*
Warm-up		
1. Jogging	1 lap	1
2. Rebound machine (60)	10	1
3. Rope skip (63)	2 minutes	1
4. Quick stop & jump (58)	5 minutes	1
5. One on one (67)	1 game	1
6. Half-court game	20 minutes	
Power Exercises		
1. Modified clean (2)	10	1
2. Squat jump (1)	10	1
Basic Exercises		
1. Squat (28)	15-15	2
2. Sit-up (26)	25-25	2
3. Heel-raise (30)	15-15	2
4. Overhead press (11)	10-10	2
5. Two-arm curl (16)	10-10	2
6. Rowing upright (13)	10-10	1
Second Half Drills		
1. Maze run (65)	1 forward, 1 backward	2
2. Endurance drill (66)	2	1

Alternate-day program

1. Jogging	1 lap	1
2. Rope skip (63)	2 minutes	1
3. Rebound machine (60)	10	1
4. Quick stop & jump (58)	5 minutes	1
5. One on one (67)	Best 2 of 3 games	1
6. Half-court game	30 minutes	1
7. Jogging	3 miles (alternating laps of jogging and running)	

IN-SEASON PROGRAM

A basketball player must undergo a terrific amount of mental and physical pressure during a playing season, so the added strain of a full weight-training program is too demanding. However, there should be some effort to maintain the strength gained through the program. The Heel Raise (30) and Squat (28) exercises should be performed at least three times a week until the beginning of the competitive season. One set of the basic exercises can also be performed. These should be done at the conclusion of the regular practice session.

After the competitive season begins there is little opportunity to weight train. The stronger players should discontinue the program. However, those players who are still weak and thin and will not play much should make an effort to get in a couple of training sessions a week. These should be done on light practice-days at the conclusion of regular practice.

PREVENTION AND REHABILITATION OF BASKETBALL INJURIES THROUGH WEIGHT TRAINING

The ankle sprain is by far the most frequent basketball injury. However, good conditioning programs and protective wrappings will prevent a large percentage of these sprains. The fact that there are many players who miss several weeks of each playing season because of sprains indicates the terrific stress placed on the joint during a game or scrimmage, and further indicates a lack of precaution or knowledge on the part of coaches and players.

Ankle Injuries — Prevention

There is probably more pressure exerted on the ankle joint than on any other joint in the body. It is not at all unusual to find a basketball player with relatively weak ankles. Preventive wrapping and taping are necessary, of course, but the support they lend the joint removes much of the stress actually needed to strengthen the muscles and tendons responsible for inverting and everting the foot. Over a long period of time the joint may become weaker if all activities are performed under a heavy "cast" of tape. Wrap the ankles before each practice, but condition the muscles responsible for movement in the ankle joint through a vigorous program of exercises and drills.

Even if the ankle is strong, it should be wrapped before the practice session by the trainer or coach. If no one is available to do this job, the coach should instruct the players carefully in the proper technique. It is much more satisfactory for them to work in pairs and wrap each other's ankles than to try to wrap their own. If the ankle has been sprained or otherwise weakened, it should be taped or strapped before participation in competitive drills. This job should always be performed by the trainer or coach.

There are a large number of exercises to strengthen the ankle joint, thereby lessening the possibility of an ankle sprain. Probably the best one is the Heel-Raise (30) exercise recommended in the training program. Sidestraddle hops with weight are also good, as are Squats (28) with the player standing on the balls of the feet. Squat Jumps (1) and Rope Skipping (63) are also good. Another exercise is to have the players walk a short distance with the feet completely inverted and the weight on the outside of the feet. All of these exercises should be practiced with no protective wrapping so that the foot muscles can be properly exercised. The ankles should be wrapped for that phase of the program which puts heavy pressure on the outside of the joint, because the large majority of sprains involve this area.

Ankle Injuries — Rehabilitation

Immediately after an ankle sprain, the joint should be wrapped with an elastic bandage over a layer of cotton. Care should be taken to see that the swelling does not make the bandage too tight. The injured ankle is elevated and cold compresses are applied for thirty to forty minutes to control internal bleeding. If the sprain is severe, weight-bearing, resistive exercises, and heat are usually not recommended until after thirty-six hours. If the sprain is not severe, non-weight-bearing exercises are started almost immediately. The exact time to start and the dosage should be determined by the team physician.

When rehabilitation exercises are indicated, the program usually follows this sequence:

1. Sitting on a table with the leg straight and flexing, extending, inverting, and everting the foot; frequently, whirlpool baths are recommended with the player exercising the ankle during the last few minutes of the bath
2. Sitting on a table with the knee flexed and performing the same exercises
3. Standing on the floor and walking around

4. Standing on the toes; later, doing Heel-Raises (30) with no weight
5. Using special apparatus. An iron shoe should be strapped on the ankle; sitting on the edge of the table with the foot hanging down, the ankle should be flexed, extended, inverted, and everted; weight should gradually be added to the shoe

In addition to the exercises previously mentioned, the exercises recommended for the prevention of ankle injuries should be used. Jogging and sprinting are also good foot exercises. If the climate is warm, running barefooted on a soft surface such as a sandy beach is an excellent foot exercise.

SELECTED REFERENCES

DeLorme, Thomas L., and Arthur L. Watkins, *Progressive Resistive Exercise.* New York: Appleton-Century-Crofts, Inc., 1951.

Morehouse, Laurence E., and Philip J. Rasch, *Scientific Basis of Athletic Training.* Philadelphia: W. B. Saunders Company, 1958.

Pinholster, Garland F., *Encyclopedia of Basketball Drills.* Englewood Cliffs, N.J.: Prentice-Hall, Inc., 1960.

Quigley, Thomas B., ed., *Sports Injuries.* The American Journal of Surgery, Inc., 1959.

Rupp, Adolph F., *Rupp's Championship Basketball.* Englewood Cliffs, N.J.: Prentice-Hall, Inc., 1958.

Sharman, Bill, *Sharman on Basketball Shooting.* Englewood Cliffs, N.J.: Prentice-Hall, Inc., 1965.

Watts, Stan, *Developing an Offensive Attack in Basketball.* Englewood Cliffs, N.J.: Prentice-Hall, Inc., 1959.

Wilkes, Glenn, *Men's Basketball.* Dubuque, Iowa: W. C. Brown Co., 1967.

8

WEIGHT TRAINING
IN FOOTBALL

Only a few years ago, college and professional football stars who trained with weights were considered an oddity. Today, they are commonplace. The value of weight training for football players has been proven many times in recent years, and the success of some of the nation's outstanding players and teams has been attributed to the strength and power gained through lifting weights.

The biggest boon to weight training for football players resulted from the achievements of the 1958 Louisiana State University football team, and particularly their star halfback, Billy Cannon. Picked to finish ninth in the Southeastern Conference, the Tigers completed an undefeated season and won the mythical National Championship. They again won their conference championship in 1959, and Cannon won the Heisman Trophy as the outstanding collegiate player of the year. These facts are significant because many of the L.S.U. players trained with weights, and Cannon, because of his weight-lifting feats, was hailed by at least one weight expert as "the strongest football player in America."[1] Weight training has been credited with much of the success of Billy Cannon and the L.S.U. Tigers.

Countless other football players have used weight training to improve their strength and power and many high schools and colleges have trained their entire squads with weights and have experienced outstanding results.

Training with weights yields the most dramatic results when used by high school teams. The probable reason is that weight training helps high school players develop muscular bodies at a stage in their lives when they are very conscious of their appearance and are very eager to improve it. As so often is the

[1] Ace Higgins, "Football's Weightlifting All-American," *Strength and Health* (November 1959), p. 34.

case in building a house, it is much easier to build a new one than it is to rebuild one that has been damaged or is in a run-down condition. The same is true in building the body. High school boys seem to respond a little more quickly to a football weight program because their bodies are still growing naturally. In college the freshmen usually realize the greatest improvement, primarily because they too are growing and maturing more rapidly.

Football provides the player with a greater opportunity than most sports for gains in strength. The leg and back muscles meet stiff resistance as the body drives into an opponent to block or tackle, or as it drives into a heavy blocking sled. The shoulder muscles are resisted in the shoulder or drive block and the arms are somewhat overloaded in tackling. This is hardly sufficient for maximum strength gains, but it might be satisfactory if it lasted over a period of time longer than sixteen to eighteen weeks (counting spring practice) of the fifty-two weeks in a year. Strength and power necessary to win football games are not developed and maintained in one-third of a year. An off-season and pre-season program of training is needed for maintaining body strength and power and for additional development of the body.

There are many college-age boys who have played football all of their lives but who are still relatively weak in vital body areas, primarily the arm, shoulder, and abdominal regions. In studies conducted at Wake Forest, we have found year after year freshman linemen who cannot chin themselves more than once. This is not nearly as unusual as it should be. Other schools, I am told, find the same to be true. If football games are to be won with these boys they must be hardened and strengthened to such a degree that they can at least handle their body weight adequately.

Many traits go into molding a winning football player. Desire is probably the most important, speed the second most important. Both are inherent abilities that cannot usually be greatly improved. Strength is the third most important, not because it isn't as necessary as the others, but because it can be increased many times by a player who has the desire.

Weight training will not assure a winning team if the players don't really have the desire to play. It accomplishes amazing results, however, with those players who have the desire for contact. They will jump at the opportunity to improve their ability. They are the leaders in an off-season weight-training program. A football player must be willing to extend himself to the maximum limit of his ability. Supreme effort must be habitual in weight training if progress is expected. In this respect the two are compatible and the best players excel and lead in both. The best weight trainees will usually be the best football players.

DISCUSSION OF SKILLS

Although there are countless skills in football, the five basic ones which are peculiar to the game and which can be improved by additional strength are blocking, tackling, running, passing, and kicking. The skills of running and kicking are important features of other games as well, but are performed somewhat differently in football.

Each basic football skill can be improved significantly through weight training and conditioning. Proper blocking and tackling should be learned by every player. Both skills require a quick burst of power (strength and speed). Therefore, if strength is greatly improved, each can be improved accordingly. Running also requires a quick burst of power and usually ends in physical contact requiring the runner to drive into an opponent. Because so often the runner must run with power against stiff resistance, this skill can probably be improved more in football than in any other sport. The other two skills — passing and kicking — require a special skill and technique. Once the skills are mastered, however, additional strength can be used to great advantage. The muscular actions of each of the five basic skills are described in the following pages in order to assist the reader in designing a weight program that will provide maximum improvements in the desired skills.

Blocking

There are many variations or types of blocks, each serving a definite purpose. The most important block a lineman must master, however, is the straight shoulder block, where one man is expected to nullify the efforts of the defensive man. No blocking technique can be substituted for this block and no lineman can hope for success without perfecting it.

In order to perform the block effectively, the player must assume a stance that will enable him to explode powerfully, beating the opponent to the punch. The best stance for delivering such a blow and for maintaining the stability needed for lateral movement should meet the following five requirements: (1) The feet should be approximately shoulder-width apart (the insides of the feet under the armpits) with the toes pointing straight ahead and the heels elevated. The feet are staggered so that if the right arm is down, the toe of the right foot is no farther back than the heel of the left foot. (2) The knees should be in line with the feet, flexed and turned in slightly. (3) The hips, shoulders, and head are all on the same plane, parallel to the ground, the shoulders squared and the head up enough to see the opponent's crotch. There is flexion at the hip, knee, and ankle joints and slight extension in the neck as the body is coiled in the most advantageous striking position. (4) The right arm should extend to the ground just inside the right knee and perpendicular to the line of scrimmage. The fingers are extended (bridged) to hold the weight. The left arm is flexed at the elbow, the forearm resting on the left knee parallel to the ground, with the fist closed. (5) The weight should be distributed so that one-third of the weight is on the right hand and two-thirds equally distributed on the balls of the feet. If both arms are extended to the ground, the weight should be distributed so that one-third of the weight is on the hands.

At the snap, the blocker fires across the line and drives the forehead into he crotch of the opponent. At the instant of contact there should be a powerful extension of the neck, lower back, and legs as the blocker attempts to lift his opponent. One arm comes to chest level as that forearm is raised as an extension of the shoulder blocking surface. The arm is winged at the shoulder and completely flexed at the elbow as the fist is held against the chest. The other arm is free and extends down as the hand seeks the ground to insure a low base and to keep from falling down and losing contact. The lifting action of the extensor muscles of the neck enables the blocker to keep his hips low and to maintain the power generated in the legs. As contact is made, the blocker slides the head to one side of the defender and takes him the desired direction, the legs churning with short, driving steps.

The muscles of the trunk and legs furnish the power in executing the block, the arms performing an action of support and balance. The initial thrust is delivered by the extensor muscles of the legs, and as contact is made the neck and low back extensors are brought vigorously into play to provide the lifting action. Muscle groups that need special attention are the neck extensors (sacrospinalis, splenius, semispinalis), knee extensors (quadriceps femoris), and the plantar flexors of the ankle (soleus, gastrocnemius). In performing the churning leg action, the legs recover quickly and powerfully; therefore, a proportionate amount of time must be devoted to the development of the flexor muscles of the hips (tensor fasciae latae, pectineus, iliopsoas) and knees (hamstrings) and the dorsal flexors of the ankle (tibialis anterior, peroneus tertius). The abductors of the shoulders (deltoid) also need special attention. These muscles not only maintain the arm in the blocking position, but also provide a cushion for protection of the shoulder joint.

Tackling

Tackling is often thought of as a shoulder block in which the tackler is allowed to use his hands and arms, usually to grasp the runner immediately after head and shoulder contact is made. Tackling technique is not considered as important as other phases of football. Several outstanding college coaches have said that tackling is only 25 percent technique or form and 75 percent desire. Increased strength and power will enhance both characteristics.

Speed and anticipation are important elements in getting into a tackling position. Immediately before launching the tackle the feet are apart, with the legs coiled, back straight, neck bowed, head up, and eyes on the target. Maneuverability is best when the feet are widened so that they are at least shoulder-width apart when the weight is carried low in a crouched position and when the stride is shortened.

The head is aimed at the mid-section of the runner to lessen the margin of error, but contact is usually made with one shoulder by dipping under the runner in a trajectory that is low and up. The tackle is launched, as is the shoulder block, with a powerful extension of the lower back and legs. As the tackle is made, the arms are carried forward, and as contact is made with the shoulder, the arms are wrapped around the runner's legs, lifting and pulling them against the chest. The head should remain up, causing contact to be on the top and front of the shoulder. Follow-through is important because it may save a first down or at least post the runner for the second man to drive him backwards. The leg drive is continuous.

As in the block, the muscles of the legs and trunk furnish the power in performing the tackle. The extensor muscles of the legs and back are brought into powerful action as the contact is made with the shoulders. Other muscle groups indicated in blocking are equally important in tackling. In addition, it is noted that the flexors of the arms (biceps, brachialis) and hands (flexor carpi group) need additional strength so that the runner may be grasped and carried to the ground.

Angle and open-field tackling probably require more speed and body control, but not as much power and desire as the head-on tackle. All are necessary phases of the game, however, in which desire for contact is mandatory.

Running

The football runner differs in certain fundamentals from the track sprinter discussed in Chapter 10. Because the runner in football usually maneuvers in a congested area, he must be prepared to move laterally and to protect or react to contact from the front or from either side. In order to do this he must: (1) run with a wider base than the track man; (2) run with a slight toe-out while in the maneuvering area; and (3) run with short, digging, pawing steps, never fully extending the knees. The wider base and toe-out enable him to maneuver better, while the shorter steps enable him to run under controlled speed, stopping and starting more quickly. By running with the knees partially flexed, he is less vulnerable to a tackle or block and is in better maneuvering position because of a lower center of gravity. If straight-ahead power is desired over maneuverability, the short, digging steps should be continued, but "the center of gravity should be thrown lower and farther forward,"[2] giving him greater hitting force and, consequently, less chance of being thrown back.

If the runner breaks from the congested area he should lengthen his stride and in so doing narrow the base and lift his center of gravity in such a way that his stride resembles that of the track sprinter. If his running area is reduced and maneuverability again becomes important, he must be able to immediately resume running under controlled speed with the wider base and shorter steps.

Even though running in football is different in some respects from that of the track sprinter, the driving force is the same in both: the extensors of the hip

[2] John W. Bunn, *Scientific Principles of Coaching.* Englewood Cliffs, N.J.: Prentice-Hall, Inc., (1955), p. 172.

(gluteus maximus) and knee (quadriceps femoris) and the plantar flexors of the ankle (soleus, gastrocnemius). These muscles must be developed for stength and speed; therefore, it is important to train them with both objectives in mind. In order to train for better lateral movement, it is also necessary to concentrate the resistive exercises in the thigh adductors (adductors, gracilis) and abductors (gluteus medius). It is especially important to strengthen and stretch the adductor muscles during early-season drills in order to lessen the likelihood of groin pulls.

Some track men who weight train lift light weights for a great number of very rapid repetitions, reportedly to guard against adding bulk to the thigh- and calf-muscle groups. A football player, however, will usually find any increase in leg size a definite asset. An increase in speed *and* strength is very desirable for both groups, but the football player must generate explosive power against the resistance of the opposition on each play. The track sprinter has no such opposition. Therefore, the football player should train for this skill by performing heavy lifts for a small number of repetitions to insure maximum strength gains and by using lighter weights a larger number of repetitions for maximum speed gains.

Track runners have found it advantageous to develop the muscles of the lower back and the arms and shoulders. It is even more important for the runner in football to develop arm, shoulder, and lower back strength because most sprints end in a block or a tackle.

In few instances does the player's run carry him more than 20 or 30 yards, whether he is blocking, tackling, or carrying the ball. For this reason the football player should supplement his weight-training program with vigorous sprints of 30 to 40 yards and with agility drills that are completed before the player is fatigued. It is very important that agility drills and sprints be full-speed drills. If endurance or stamina is desired, the drills should be performed with only a short rest.

Passing

The throwing motion of the football passer is very similar to that of the baseball catcher. In the cocking motion, the body is turned sideways to the target with the feet fairly close together. The weight is shifted to the rear leg as the ball is brought to a position behind the right ear. As the pass is made, the front foot steps toward the intended target, the weight is shifted from the right to the left leg, the left arm is held out comfortably for balance, and the ball is thrown with a smooth but snaplike motion. A good follow-through toward the target assures a proper shift in weight.

Although the throwing motion is basically the same as that described in baseball, there are some slight differences. The football passer must usually stand tall in order to see over the line when passing. Because of the size and shape c the football, the passer must release the ball in such a way as to impart the proper spin to it. The motion resembles the baseball pitcher throwing a screwball, the ball rolling off the forefinger and middle finger and the palm turning out as the ball is released.

The act of passing involves a full body movement, but the power for the throw is generated by the muscles of the arm and shoulder. The horizontal flexors of the shoulder (anterior deltoid, pectoralis major, serratus anterior), the extensors of the arm (triceps), and the pronators of the forearm (pronator quadratus) are the muscles primarily responsible for strong, accurate passing. The flexor muscles of the wrist and fingers impart the final impetus. Special emphasis should be placed on the development of each of these muscle groups for stronger, more accurate throwing.

Kicking

A ball is usually kicked in one of two methods: the punt or the place kick. The fundamentals are similar for each method, though the punt sends the ball spiraling from the foot, whereas the place kick produces an end-over-end movement. For successful achievement, both methods require a high degree of coordination, long hours of practice, and powerful legs.

The stance for the punt is a heel and toe alignment, with the kicking foot forward and the feet slightly spread. The body is in a semi-crouched position, so that a poor snap from center can be better fielded. The first step is a short one by the kicking leg, followed by a full step with the other leg. The kicking foot is then driven forward, with the toes depressed, the leg extending forcefully at the knee as contact is made with the ball. The follow-through is completed by extending the kicking foot forward toward the target and bringing it back down in the same plane. The other foot remains firmly planted on the ground so that good balance can be maintained. The eyes should watch the ball until it is kicked and the body should move forward throughout, though at impact the body actually is leaning slightly away from the ball. For maximum distance and minimum kicking error under normal conditions, the ball should leave the foot at an angle of approximately 45 degrees and should be dropped as short a distance as possible, contact being made below the knee height.

The fundamentals of the place kick are very similar to those of the punt. However, the place kick is different in that the kicking foot is held at almost a right angle to the leg and is held rigid at the instant it contacts the ball to prevent any recoil action. The steps are almost the same as for the punt, the kicking foot stepping first with the other foot hitting about two-and-a-half inches to the side of and behind the ball. The foot drives through the ball with a powerful leg snap, the knee locking in order to get a pendulum action from the hip. To assure proper follow-through, the kicker keeps his head down and his body bent forward until the kicking foot hits the ground again.

The muscles of the legs furnish the power in performing the punt and the place kick. The hip flexors (iliopsoas, tensor fasciae latae) contract vigorously to bring the kicking leg forward, but the powerful contraction of the extensors of the knee (quadriceps femoris) are responsible for the leg snap necessary for good kicking. In the punt, the plantar flexors of the foot (gastrocnemius, soleus) contract to hold the foot rigidly in position.

Kickers should be especially careful to maintain balance in the strength of the leg muscles. Though primary emphasis should be on the development of the hip flexors and knee extensors, the extensors of the hip (gluteus maximus) and the knee flexors (hamstrings) should not be neglected. Improper muscle balance often leads to pulled hamstring muscles. Each workout should be preceded by a period of stretching and loosening exercises.

SUPPLEMENTARY EXERCISES AND DRILLS

Books of football drills have been written for the purpose of improving football skills. Only a few that should be used to supplement the weight-training program are included in this chapter. These drills are described so that a player can apply the strength and power he will derive from a weight-training program to the game of football by practicing the related skills. As a rule, they should be done on alternate days of a pre-season or off-season program of weight training by one or two, or a small group of players. No team drills are described because many conferences do not allow off-season football practice.

If time or coaching personnel are limited or restricted on the alternate days, so that only a few of the drills can be performed, it is recommended that the program consist entirely of the speed and agility drills. The conditioning drills should be conducted during the pre-season practice and occasionally during the playing season. Kicking and passing drills are available in books on football drills, and should be studied extensively by players who wish to become skilled in these specialties.

Speed and Agility Drills

68. Sprints

The starting position is a good offensive stance with the body weight shifted slightly forward. The player should fire out and sprint for 40 yards, slow down gradually and walk for 40 yards. There should be a concentration on a quick start followed by a burst of speed. Players should be timed on this drill and should race by positions in order to maintain competition and enthusiasm. They should not use it if they are improperly warmed up or after they are fatigued. Start with a snap count and, if timing, start the watch on the first reaction of the player in order to reduce the margin of error in comparing scores Occasionally get comparative times on verbal and visual signals also.

69.   Maze run (football)

Place four markers (i.e., blocking dummies) as shown in the illustration. A properly marked football field makes placing the standards an easy task. The course should be run both forward and backward. Encourage the players, in going forward, to cut around the standards, not circle them. In going through backward, the players should simulate pass defense, keeping their eyes on the starting mark (i.e., passer) and picking up the standards using peripheral vision. This drill is good for linemen as well as backs, because agility and speed are desirable outcomes. They can be timed separately on running forward, backward, forward and backward together, or on running forward through the maze and returning.

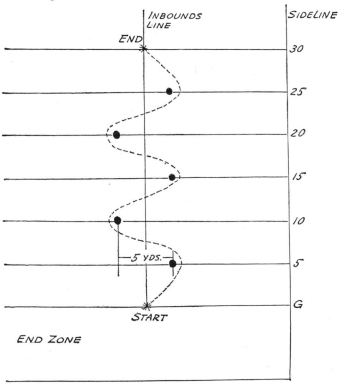

Figure 68. Maze Run, Football

70.   Around the block

This drill teaches quick forward, lateral, and backward movements. Place four markers as shown in the illustration. From a good offensive stance, run forward to the first marker, go left using a crossover step to the second marker, n backward to the third marker, and shuffle sideward to the right to the finish . The stop watch is an excellent motivator in this drill. Strive for speed.

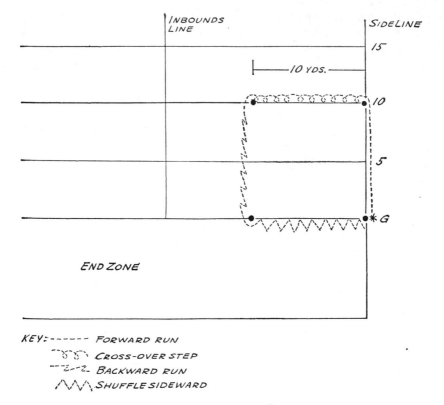

INBOUNDS LINE   SIDELINE

Figure 69. Around the Block

71. Dumbbell run

Hold a 25-pound dumbbell in each hand and start from a standing position. Sprint for a distance of 30 yards, turn around and sprint back. The drill may be varied by gradually increasing the weight of the dumbbells and by running relays.

72. Grass drill

Even though this drill is usually used as a conditioning drill, it is excellent for developing agility and for hardening the body. Any number of players may participate, with one setting the pace. Give the drills only on a dry grass area. Begin by using a stationary run, concentrating on a high knee lift and running on the toes. At the command, "front," quickly fall to the ground, face down, using the hands to absorb some of the fall, but taking a good part of it with the stomach. On the command "up," return quickly to running in place. On the command "back," bend forward and roll back on the seat and then the back. On the command "right," roll over one complete revolution to the right, and on the command "left," roll over a complete revolution to the left. Follow any squence of the commands, front, back, right, left, inserting any others you might thir up. In order to make this an effective agility drill, it is recommended that it be limited to one minute.

73. Crab

This drill is excellent for teaching linemen to move quickly and low, as after being knocked down by a block. Assume the crab position; head up, back straight, buttocks down, feet spread shoulder-width, and knees bent and about two inches off the turf. Using short, quick steps, execute the following movements on verbal or visual signals: forward, back, right, and left.

74. Forward and shoulder rolls

This is a good drill for teaching a player how to break a fall and make a quick recovery into a hitting position. Forward momentum is necessary for proper execution. In the forward roll, the initial shock is taken by the hands and as the body follows, the head is tucked under and the weight is caught on the back of the neck and shoulders. Tuck the knees and flex at the hips and trunk to make the roll, recovering to a hitting position.

The shoulder roll is fundamentally the same except that the original shock is received on the back of either the right or left shoulder. If the call is "right," the right arm is pulled in and the right shoulder is down as the roll is executed on that side. The opposite is true for the left side.

75. Rope skip

One of the very best drills for agility and coordination is rope-skipping. Players should be encouraged to practice skipping at least three times a week during the entire off-season. Heavier players should skip a few minutes every day.

Conditioning Drills

76. Strides

This is an excellent drill for stretching the groin and hamstring muscles of the leg. Starting from a three-point stance, the player sprints 10 to 20 yards, lengthening the stride with each step until he is actually taking a long leap with each step. Continue the strides for 30 yards before easing off and jogging for 10 to 15 yards. Assume the three-point stance and repeat. Warm up properly before using this drill.

77. Five more

Five more is a combination agility and endurance exercise. Have the player take a three-point stance on the goal line facing upfield. Sprint to the five-yard line and return to the goal line. Without stopping, sprint to the ten-yard line and return to the goal line; then to the fifteen, etc. Continue at top speed to work up the field as far as possible, returning to the goal line each time. The further the player can work upfield at top speed, the better his physical condition.

78. Cross-country run

One of the most gruelling conditioning drills in sports is the cross-country run. However, the only way to build up the wind for football is by running relatively long distances. Football demands sprint-type running, but distance running is also necessary in order to develop the degree of endurance needed to play a large part of a game. A lot of both is indicated. The cross-country run should cover all kinds of terrain, including hills, stadium steps, etc. The players should be timed and encouraged to run against the stop watch. This drill is especially valuable during the six weeks before official practice begins.

79. Conditioning games

Any game that requires a lot of running and has no body contact is a good game for off-season conditioning. Four games we have seen used are handball, touch football, flicker ball, and speedball. Be certain to modify the rules so that there is absolutely no contact. Conditioning games give the players an opportunity to compete against each other and add needed variety to the program. These games are especially valuable during the off-season lifting program. It is imperative that the games be highly competitive. Reward the winners and penalize the losers. Use tournaments of all types.

80. Quadriceps strengthener

The Bench Technique, developed by Klein[3] at the University of Texas for improving the strength and driving power of the leg, is also probably the most effective method to prevent knee injuries. The program outlined below is patterned after that used by Klein and makes use of the bench illustrated in Figure 7. The player should sit on the bench with his feet under the adjustable bar and the back of the knee 2 to 3 inches above the front edge of the bench. By forcefully contracting the quadriceps muscles, the legs are straightened and the body raised perpendicularly from the bench. Perform the exercise at such a speed that the leg extension and the return to the starting position require approximately three seconds. Two sets should be performed each exercise period with at least one minute rest between them. The players should work up to a minimum of fifty repetitions in each set before regular outdoor practice begins.

Sample program

First Week	Sets	Repetitions
First day	One	15
	Two	20
Second day	One	20
	Two	25
Third day	One	20
	Two	30
Second Week		
First day	One	25
	Two	30

[3] Karl K. Klein, "The Bench Technique of Exercise — A Mass Method for Increasing Leg Driving Power, Preventive Conditioning, and Reduction of Knee Injury Potential in Athletics," *Texas Coach* (February 1961).

Second day	One	30
	Two	35
Third day	One	30
	Two	40

Third Week

First day	One	35
	Two	40
Second day	One	40
	Two	45
Third day	One	40
	Two	50

OFF-SEASON PROGRAM

The off-season weight-training program should last at least three months and preferably longer. The first month should be devoted to a basic program of exercises in which the primary emphasis should be on improvement of general body condition and muscle tone. Little or no attempt should be made to increase the weight loads until the third or fourth week. The program should contain several lifts that require a full body movement, but the majority of the exercises should be basic and simple. The program suggested in this chapter can be shortened by omitting certain lifts. However, the Bench Press, Squat, and Dead Lift exercises are the heart of the football program and should not be shortened.

During the second and third months the training tempo is increased. The players should go up on their weight loads any time they can complete ten repetitions on the second set. At least once every two weeks the repetitions should be cut to five, three, and one, and heavier weights lifted. The quadriceps bench should be used by all players during the off-season until they can complete two sets of knee extensors for fifty repetitions. If a quadriceps bench is not available, three extra sets of squats should be performed. The Neck Exercises (8, 9) are replaced by the Wrestler's Bridge (10), and the Dead Lift, Straight Legs (25) is replaced by the Dead Lift (29). During the latter stages of the program, the Dumbbell Run (71), Squat Jump (1), Straight-Arm Pullover (23), and the Heel-Raise (30) should be used occasionally to provide variety. It is also a good idea to increase the number of repetitions in the power exercises from ten to twelve as strength and power increase and to increase the weight load occasionally as long as the player can perform the lift with an explosive action.

The lifting program is the same for linemen, backs, kickers, and passers. Heavier players should be encouraged to participate in a very rigorous alternate-day program.

Lifting Program

Exercise	Repetitions	Sets
Warm-up		
1. Jogging	1 lap	1
2. Rope skip	1 minute	1
3. Squat thrust	10	1
4. Alternate toe touches	10	1
Power Exercises		
1. Modified clean (2)	10	1
2. Power press (4)	10	1
3. Power curl (3)	10	1
4. Quadriceps bench (80)	See Drill (80)	2
5. Squat jump (1)	10	1
Basic Exercises		
1. Squat (28)	15-15	2
2. Bench press (22)	10-10	2
3. Sit-ups (26)	25-maximum to 100	2
4. Overhead press (11)	10-10	2
5. Two-arm curl (16)	10-10	2
6. Dead lift, straight legs (25)*	15-15	2
7. Rowing upright (13)	10-10	2
8. Neck exercises (8,9)**	2 (holding each 7 seconds)	1

Alternate-day Program

The success of a football weight program can be greatly enhanced with a well-organized and properly supervised alternate-day program. The drills recommended in this program are primarily speed and agility drills that may be performed indoors as well as outdoors with a minimum amount of planning. During the first day of the program the players should be timed on the Maze Run (69), Around the Block (70) and the Sprints (68). They should be periodically timed thereafter and made aware of their scores on the tests and encouraged to beat them. It is very important that the heavier players participate in such a program a minimum of three days a week and it is recommended that *all* players participate in this program at least two days of the week. Rope-Skipping (75) can be done a few minutes each day.

It is necessary to add variety to the alternate-day program if interest is to be maintained. This is done by having the players race against each other or

*Change to Dead Lift (29) after one month.
**Change to Wrestler's Bridge (10) after one month.

against the stop watch. Another excellent method is to supplement the program with one of the Conditioning Games (79). Organizing tournaments also helps to engender enthusiasm.

Alternate-day program

Exercise	Repetitions	Sets
1. Jogging	1 lap	1
2. Grass drill (72)	1 minute	1
3. Around the block (70)	1 forward	1
4. Crab (73)	1 minute	1
5. Maze run (69)	1 forward, 1 backward, 1 forward and return	1
6. Sprints (68)	5	1

Power Rack Program (Hold each exercise approximately seven seconds)

1. Heel-raise (38)
2. Overhead press (34)
3. Curl (33)
4. Bench press (37)
5. Upright rowing (35)
6. Dead lift (36)

PRE-SEASON PROGRAM

The pre-season training program should be designed to so condition the players through a variety of lifting exercises and football drills that they will be able to go at top speed on the first day of practice, losing a minimum amount of time to sore muscles. It should last about six weeks and should not go beyond the first official practice period.

The lifting program should approximate the off-season program, the changes from the Neck Exercises to the Wrestler's Bridge and the Dead Lift, Straight Legs to the Dead Lift coming after approximately three weeks.

The warm-up phase of the program differs from that of the off-season program in that every effort should be made to have the players participate in speed and conditioning drills during the pre-season program. During the first three weeks the emphasis is primarily on speed drills. A suggested warm-up is:

Exercise	Repetitions
1. Jogging	1 lap
2. Sprints (68)	5
3. Strides (76)	5
4. Sit-ups (26)	25
5. Rope skip (75)	1 minute

During the last three weeks conditioning type drills such as Five More (77) should be included in the warm-up program and the amount of jogging increased. All of the warm-up drills should be done outdoors if the weather permits so that the legs may be properly conditioned to the ground. If the weather does not permit, the drills should be adapted to the gymnasium.

Kickers and passers should use appropriate drills to train for their specialties before they participate in the routine program. Success in the performance of the skills is dependent on a great amount of off-season and pre-season practice, and those players who handle these duties for their teams will have to spend a great deal of extra time on the practice field if they expect to perfect them.

Alternate-day Program

The pre-season alternate-day program should emphasize sprinting and distance running. Agility drills should also be included, especially for the linemen and heavier players. The suggested program outlined below should be varied from day to day by introducing a variety of conditioning games, by increasing the distance of the cross-country run to two or three miles, by substituting other drills, and by having plenty of good competition in the drills, the boys competing against each other or against the watch.

Alternate-day program

Exercise	Repetitions
1. Jogging	2 laps
2. Strides (76)	5
3. Sprints (68)	2 lengths of field
4. Five more (77)	Maximum at top speed
5. Grass drill (72)	1 minute
6. Rope skip (75)	1–2 minutes
7. Conditioning game (79)	
8. Cross-country run (78)	

Power Rack Program
(Hold each exercise approximately seven seconds)
1. Heel-raise (38)
2. Overhead press (34)
3. Curl (33)
4. Bench press (37)
5. Upright rowing (35)
6. Dead lift (36)

IN-SEASON PROGRAM

During the playing season, one lifting session a week is usually sufficient to maintain strength previously gained through a weight program. It is not advisable to start a player on a lifting program during the season unless an injury has weakened his general strength. The best day to lift is usually the second day after game day and before the heavy work begins for the following week's game.

The program should consist of those lifts which exercise the major muscle groups of the body and particularly those muscles that are used most in running, blocking, and tackling. Two sets of each exercise should be sufficient if a boy is getting to play regularly and is staying in top shape. Little attempt should be made to increase the weight loads. The first set should be performed with approximately one-half the maximum weight load and the second set with three-quarters the maximum load. The entire program should take only thirty to forty minutes if the players hustle through it.

Lifting program

Exercise	Repetitions	Sets
Warm-up		
1. Jogging	1 lap	1
2. Squat thrust	10	1
3. Alternate toe touches	10	1
Power Exercises		
1. Power press (4)	10	1
2. Power curl (3)	10	1
3. Quadriceps strengthener (80)	50	2
Basic Exercises		
1. Overhead press (11)	10–8	2
2. Two-arm curl (16)	10–8	2
3. Dead lift, straight legs (25)	10–8	2
4. Sit-up (26)	25	1
5. Bench press (22)	10–8	2
6. Squat (28)	12–10	2

PREVENTION AND REHABILITATION OF FOOTBALL INJURIES THROUGH WEIGHT TRAINING

The knee and the shoulder are two of the weakest joints in the body. They are also two of the most vulnerable to injury in the game of football. The shoulder pad has eliminated a large percentage of shoulder injuries, but so far, an adequate safeguard for the knee has not been devised. The strength of both joints can be greatly improved through weight training, and the frequency of injuries sharply reduced.

Knee Injuries — Prevention

Knee injuries shorten the careers of probably more high school and college football players than any other type of injury, and many former players still suffer from "football knees" sustained twenty to thirty years ago. A large percentage of these injuries could have been avoided and many players could have completely recovered had they understood the value of resistive exercise with weights. Football coaches make a terrible mistake if they don't have their players participate in a thorough program of exercises for the knees before each season and each spring practice begins. Too often a rash of knee injuries is blamed on improper shoes, poor turf, clipping, or just bad luck. These are usually contributing factors, but the coach alone is to blame if he hasn't done all in his power to influence his players to strengthen the quadricep and hamstring muscle groups that support and protect the knee joint.

Many coaches feel that in running, blocking, and tackling, the muscles surrounding the knee are strengthened sufficiently to prevent injury to that joint. However, this logic can't be supported. In actual practice, football players who begin resistive exercises of the quadriceps muscle at the close of a season, realize rapid gains in strength. We have even found some players who have lost some quadricep strength during a playing season, indicating a possible need for an in-season program of resistive exercises for the knees, especially for those players who aren't playing much.

Most football coaches have abandoned the full squat, the duck walk, and other similar exercises because of the possibility that the ligaments around the knee might be stretched. Actually, there is no position or movement in football that requires a player to fully flex the knees. Therefore, even though it is a certainty that many players can perform the full squat with no ill effects, they do not contribute anything to the knee joint and should be omitted from the program.

A very successful method to prevent knee injury is to use the program outlined in Drill 80. Such a program develops the quadriceps muscle group to such a degree that the knee joint is much more stable and the likelihood of knee injuries is sharply reduced. This muscle group should be well defined when the leg is fully extended and should be so well developed that the medial portion above the knee (vastus medialis) literally bulges. Some authorities say that the hamstring muscles behind the knee are also strengthened because they extend the knee during the final few degrees if the foot is in contact with the ground.

Another method to strengthen the quadriceps is through the use of the knee flexor-extensor table or through other commercial knee strengtheners that operate on the same principle. The flexor-extensor table (see Figure 5) is designed so that the player can sit with the legs hanging from the end with the top of the feet under the weighted bar. When the legs extend at the knee the feet lift the bar, and as the legs relax and bend the bar returns to its original position. College football players should be able to extend 100 pounds eight to ten repetitions with each leg. High school players won't be able to handle quite as much weight, but should work toward that goal.

Although not as important to knee stability, it is important also to develop the hamstring muscle group behind the knee. This can be done best on the flexor-extensor table. Lying face down, hook the back of the ankles under the top support and flex the legs at the knee. Start with light weight and graduate the resistance until the hamstring strength has been developed to at least within 55-60 percent of the quadriceps. Use the same two-set program of ten, 10 repetitions, for development of the hamstring and quadriceps muscle groups.

Either program of resistive exercises mentioned above should be used in conjunction with a complete lifting program in which the Squat and Dead Lift exercises are an important part. Other leg exercises, such as the Heel-Raises, are valuable exercises that can be used to advantage at times to supplement the knee-strengthening program.

Knee Injuries — Rehabilitation

Resistive exercises are needed to restore knee stability after an operation. A post-operative program of exercises should be under the supervision of a trained orthopedist and the resistive exercises are only a basic part of a sound rehabilitation program. However, there are many instances in which boys, especially in high schools, have undergone knee operations and their entire post-operative program consisted of tying some sandbags on the foot of the injured leg and exercising it. Rehabilitation from a knee operation is a delicate procedure and should be outlined step by step by the surgeon. The program of exercises described in the following paragraph is a general description of the type of program that is often prescribed.

As a rule, the first step after the actual pain of the operation has subsided is quadriceps setting exercises, which consist merely of contracting or tensing the quadriceps muscle. Soon thereafter, straight leg-raising exercises are added, the only movement being flexion at the hip joint. These are usually continued until the stitches are removed, whereupon nonresisted knee flexion and extension exercises are begun. These are continued for two to three weeks before weight is added. If using the flexor-extensor table, begin by using the resistance of the bar only. When three sets of ten can be performed, add weight when the third set can be performed for ten repetitions. The knee should regain its normal strength and range of motion within two to three months. It is necessary to overdevelop the muscles in order to compensate for any ligament weakness due to injury.

After each program, the leg should be held in an extended position for two or three minutes by flexing the quadriceps muscle. This helps to further tone the quadriceps and assures maximum exercise of the vastus medialis muscle which is said to be responsible for the last fifteen degrees of extension of the knee. When the muscles of the injured leg are developed beyond those of the uninjured one, it is a good indication that the knee is near normal.

For maximum stability of the knee joint, the hamstring muscle group also needs resistive exercise after surgery. The player should begin by standing on one leg and lifting the foot of the injured leg so that the knee flexes. Bend the knee only partially at first and gradually lift it to a high knee position. If the flexor-extensor table is available, have the player lie on his stomach on the table and flex the leg at the knee. Next, hook both ankles under the bar and flex the legs, bearing most of the weight with the uninjured leg. As the strength of the injured leg improves, exercise it alone, gradually increasing the weight.

An iron boot is often used for hamstring strengthening, but must be used with caution and only after the knee is well on its way to recovery. The exercise is performed by standing on a platform so the injured knee with the attached boot hangs free. Flex the leg at the knee and lower, gradually increasing the weight attached to the boot. Lying on the stomach and flexing the leg at the knee is not recommended because there is danger that the weighted boot may cause the unstable knee to flex too much or to twist or fall to either side.

The strength of the quadricep and hamstring muscle groups will usually return more quickly than the size of the muscle, but the size will return with continued work. Players who must undergo a knee operation will find it beneficial to build up the muscle groups surrounding the knee before the operation. This speeds the post-operative strength-building program considerably.

Shoulder Dislocation

While blocking or tackling, a player's arm is occasionally pulled or rotated from its very shallow socket at the shoulder joint. The pain from such an injury is severe and the recovery is slow and very seldom complete. Often the player is allowed to return to play by wearing a special harness which prevents him from lifting the arm. However, care must be taken in all activities, because once the shoulder has been dislocated, it becomes increasingly easy to do it again.

The structure of the shoulder joint is one of the weakest in the body. The joint depends almost entirely on surrounding muscles and tendons for strength. Besides holding the head of the bone in the shallow cavity of the shoulder, the muscles also help protect the joint by providing a muscular pad or cushion over the point of the shoulder.

The best way to safeguard against a shoulder dislocation in football is to develop powerful arms and shoulders. This doesn't require a special program of exercises exclusively for the shoulders. The basic football weight program is sufficient if conscientiously practiced. If the player is especially weak in the shoulder region, there are several good exercises with the barbell and dumbbells that can be added. The Lateral Raise, Standing (15), and the Straight-Arm Pullover (23) should be beneficial if included in the program.

In rehabilitating a dislocated shoulder, the physician will usually suggest exercises to rebuild the muscles surrounding the joint. These are administered after most of the pain has left, starting with the most simple exercises and progressing to fairly heavy lifts. Rehabilitation of the shoulder joint is not usually a rapid process, so it is very important that the player be patient and take one step at a time. Shoulder stability will be improved considerably, but it is extremely doubtful that it will approach its original strength.

SELECTED REFERENCES

Allen, George H., *Complete Book of Winning Football Drills.* Englewood Cliffs, N.J.: Prentice-Hall, Inc., 1959.

Baker, William A., Jr., "The Pete Dawkins Story," *Strength and Health* (December 1959), p. 36.

Biggs, Ernest R., *Conditioning for Football,* Dubuque, Iowa: W. C. Brown Co., 1968.

Dietzel, Paul F., *Coaching Football.* New York: Ronald Press Co., 1971.

McKay, John H., *Football Coaching.* New York: Ronald Press Co., 1966.

Murray, Jim, "Stan Jones, All-America Football Star," *Strength and Health* (August 1954), p. 10.

9

WEIGHT TRAINING
IN SWIMMING

Although most swimming coaches agree that competitive swimmers must have powerful muscles, there is much disagreement as to how this power should be acquired. Most coaches agree that training with weights will increase power, but many contend that the increase will be accompanied by shortened muscles and restricted joint action. Such a philosophy is similar to that of basketball coaches who don't allow their players to train with weights because they fear that they will lose their "touch"; or to that of baseball coaches who contend that weight training will so "tie up" the shoulders of a player that he won't be able to hit or throw. Such theories have recently been proven completely false through the use of sensible weight training programs.

It is true that competitive swimming requires the well-stretched and the well-developed muscle. As a matter of fact the good swimmer, even more than the basketball or baseball player, needs these qualities. The arms and legs must exert a tremendous effort again and again as they pull with a finely coordinated action and recover with maximum speed for the next stroke.

Competitive swimming and flexibility exercises have been the backbone of most training programs for many years. Creditable records were established primarily because the champions were highly skilled and well conditioned. In recent years, however, swimming records of long standing and of every description have taken an incredible beating. It isn't accidental that during the same span of years weight training and other forms of resistive exercise have been used increasingly by many of the world's best swimmers. There is good logic for this. Practicing swimming doesn't develop the muscular strength that is necessary for an individual to reach his maximum performance. The amount of overload provided by the resistance of the water is a constant factor and therefore is not sufficient for maximum strength gains. Sprint and distance swimming overload for speed and endurance respectively. Strength should be built by the much heavier overloads that can be found in weight training.

The two swimmers who probably did most to popularize weight training were Dick Cleveland and Al Wiggins of Ohio State University, both of whom set world records after vigorous weight-training periods. Both men were very good swimmers before they began weight training, but only after they had improved their muscular strength did they set swimming records.

The fact that Cleveland and Wiggins trained with weights is important to all competitive swimmers. Even more important, however, is the fact that they gave weight training a lion's share of the credit for their record-breaking performances. Wiggins went so far as to say, "I have proved that training with weights is the most beneficial thing a swimmer can do out of water."[1]

These men set the tempo for many of the current crop of record-smashing swimmers. Most of the outstanding competitive swimmers in the world today are strong and powerful athletes, and many of them acquired a large part of this strength by training regularly with weights as they developed their swimming skill. Perhaps the most famous is Dr. James Counsilman, head swimming coach at Indiana, who has trained a large number of collegiate and Olympic champions by combining weight training and other forms of resistive exercise with swimming programs. In recent years Dr. Counsilman has made extensive use of isokinetic equipment.

DISCUSSION OF SKILLS

The competitive swimmer's success is influenced by many factors. Probably the most important one is his physical make-up. He must have powerful muscles in almost all regions of the body; wrists, arms, shoulders, back, abdomen, legs, and ankles. The joints must be very flexible with a large range of motion. The muscles must also be finely controlled by the swimmer, and his coordinated movement in performing a stroke, especially during the pulling phase, must be flawless.

Probably the second most important factor is speed. It is impossible really to separate speed from strength, because the faster one swims the greater the resistance of the water becomes; and the greater this resistance becomes the greater is the demand for strength. No degree of success can be attained if the muscles can't exert explosive bursts of power in both the arm pull and the leg kick. This power is achieved through a proportional increase of strength and speed.

[1] Bob Hoffman, *Better Athletes Through Weight Training* York, Pa.: Strength and Health Publishing Company, (1959), p. 270.

The third factor is desire. Just as in any sport, the best swimmer has to endure the terrific pain of fatigue and push past this barrier to reach a peak of physical condition. Only those who have the burning desire to be champions and who are willing to pay the price of extremely hard conditioning programs will be successful, regardless of their physical qualifications.

The competitive strokes have evolved over a period of many years, with almost constant improvements in stroke techniques and conditioning and training methods. The four strokes used in modern competitive swimming are the free style (front crawl), back crawl, breast stroke, and butterfly stroke. Skills in some other sports require only an average amount of strength, but performance of these swimming skills requires a maximum amount of muscular strength and power. Every method must be employed to improve this power.

Only the four competitive strokes are analyzed in this chapter. There are skills other than stroking to be learned for competitive swimming. For example, starting and turning are extremely important and considerable effort should be made to improve the performance of these skills. Because the swimmer who improves his strength and performance in any of the four strokes should also be improving the other skills, only these strokes are discussed and analyzed for weight training.

Divers also can find weight training beneficial. No attempt has been made to analyze the many complex dives because a diver must have excellent muscular development in all body regions. A diver should use a general weight program concentrating only on muscle groups that are particularly weak. A program similar to that of the pole vaulter suggested in Chapter 10 should prove beneficial.

Free Style

In swimming the shorter free style races the swimmer carries his head with the face in the water, the water line striking between the eyes and the hairline depending on the buoyancy of the swimmer. The eyes are focused straight ahead and the neck is not rigid. The shoulders are raised but the upper back is slightly flexed or hunched. The rest of the trunk is parallel to the surface of the water. The legs extend behind and the kick is maintained slightly under the surface of the water.

The three important factors in the free style, or crawl stroke, are the overarm stroke, the flutter kick, and breathing.

1.   The arm stroke

The arms provide the major portion of the force in performing the free style, alternately reaching out to grab a handful of water, and pulling the body along. One arm is extended backward near the hips at the completion of the drive. The other is extended straight from the shoulder and hits the water as far out as possible, with the fingertips entering first. As it presses downward, the tip of the elbow points sideward and the pressure of the arm on the water supports the body. The faster the stroke, the greater the momentum of the swimmer, thus less support is needed. The catch takes place when the hand is 6 to 10 inches below the water surface. The catch is an inward movement of the hand and arm, in which the hand is brought back along an imaginary center line of the body. The elbow is bent to allow the swimmer to maintain the hand in this plane during the pull. As the arm reaches the hip, the hand is flexed quickly to give a final impetus to the arm stroke.

At the completion of the final push, the arm is lifted from the water in the recovery. The elbow is lifted first; then the forearm and hand should recover quickly and effortlessly. The elbow moves forward and when it is even with the head, the forearm begins to move out ahead of the elbow until the arm is completely extended again and ready for re-entry.

The timing of the arm action is such that as the catch is made with one hand the other has recovered to a position about even with the face. As the recovered arm enters the water the other is well into the pull, and at the beginning of the catch it has just recovered out of the water.

2.   **The flutter kick**

In performing the flutter kick the swimmer exerts pressure on the sole of the foot during the upward stroke and on the top of the foot during the downward. The initial movement is in the hip joint, and the motion subsequently carries down through the knee, ankle, and foot. The whiplash action of the foot provides the bulk of the propelling action for the entire leg. The width of the kick should be approximately 15 to 20 inches. Some power is obtained on the downthrust of the leg, but the emphasis for propulsion is on the upthrust, the other being more of a recovery than a propelling force. The knee should bend a bit as the knee extensors are allowed to relax slightly on the downthrust. The toes are extended and turned inward; they should not break the surface on the upward thrust. The legs perform six beats to the complete arm cycle, or three beats to each arm revolution.

3.   **Breathing**

The most common form of breathing is to inhale through the mouth above the surface and to exhale through the mouth and nose under the surface. The frequency with which breaths should be taken is a debatable question. The shorter the race, the faster the stroke, and the less often the swimmer actually breathes. In breathing, the head should not be raised, but should be rotated to the side for air and returned as quickly as possible. The chin is tucked in close to the throat as the head turns in the channel, and the mouth is opened as it clears the water. Air is taken in quickly before the mouth closes and the head returns to the water. When it is back in the center, air is expelled at once and is not taken in again before the next stroke.

Between inhalations the face should point directly ahead. In competitiv swimming it is important that the inhalation be completed as quickly as possib

If the swimmer breathes on the left side he should rotate the head to the left as the left arm passes the face. As the left hand is lifted from the water in the recovery, the head should begin the return, and by the time the left hand has recovered even with the face, the head should be in its original position. Although most swimmers breathe on only one side, there are definite advantages to breathing on both sides; in the longer races the swimmer can breathe on every third stroke. This allows him to see his opponents on both sides, thereby enabling him to swim a more intelligent race. It also enables him to breathe less often and to use the muscles on each side of the neck in a more natural coordinated movement.

The muscles of the chest, back, shoulders, and arms furnish a major portion of the power in executing the free style. In the catch, pull, and push phases of the arm stroke the major power is generated by the shoulder extensors (latissimus dorsi, pectoralis major). The forearm flexors (biceps, brachialis) contract to keep the elbow slightly flexed against the resistance of the water and forearm pronators (pronator teres, pronator quadratus) hold the arm in slight pronation. The flexor muscles of the wrist and hands contract to hold the hand in a strong position as the pull is made. These muscles need to be very powerful. The abductors and hyperextensors of the shoulder (trapezius, serratus anterior, deltoid) and the extensors of the elbow (triceps) are important in the recovery, and although their action is not heavily resisted they should be strengthened in proportion to the harder-working muscles of the arms and shoulders.

The muscles of the trunk are important in stabilizing the body and for breathing. The abdominals (rectus abdominis, obliques) and the back extensors (sacrospinalis, erector spinae) must be well-conditioned to provide this function.

The muscles of the legs provide a relatively small percentage of the propulsive force. On the downstroke the thigh flexors (iliopsoas, tensor fasciae latae) and the knee extensors (quadriceps femoris) contract. The real power of the kick is in the upstroke. The extensors of the hip and knee (hamstrings, gluteus maximus) are powerfully contracted, as are the plantar flexors (soleus, gastrocnemius) and inward rotators (tibialis posterior) of the foot.

Back Crawl

The back crawl swimmer is little different from the free styler turned over. The arms and legs move at about the same speed in both. Of course the breathing is quite different. As in the free style, the inhaling should be done through the mouth to prevent water coming into the nose, and the exhaling can be through the nose and mouth. Otherwise, the breathing rhythm is as normal as it would be in performing any vigorous activity out of water.

The body position is almost straight and as nearly close to the surface of the water as possible, with the hips just under the surface. The head is straight and the chin is tucked so that the swimmer can see his feet. The back of the head is about halfway under the water, with the bottom of the ears about even with the surface.

1. The arm stroke

Starting with the arm at the side the recovery is started by lifting the shoulder so that the arm can be brought cleanly out of the water. The elbow is bent slightly and the palm faces the water as the relaxed arm is brought back at no more than a 45-degree angle from the line of the body. The entry is made with the arm extended and the palm facing outward. Immediately after the arm enters the water the elbow bends so that when it reaches shoulder level it is bent at approximately 90 degrees. The pull continues down the side of the body, the hand remaining only 4 to 10 inches below the surface until the final push before the recovery is started.

The timing of the arm action is such that the arms are directly opposite each other in a windmill fashion. When one arm is at the thigh the other is entering the water and they maintain these relative positions.

2. The flutter kick

If a swimmer has developed a good free style kick he should have little trouble using the same basic kick in the back crawl. The movement of the hips, knees, ankles, and feet are basically the same for both strokes. The biggest difference is that in the back crawl kick the knee bend should be greater and the feet appear to break the water slightly.

In the upward thrust the knee bends and then quickly straightens as the foot whips up so that at the end of the thrust the leg is in a straight line with the body. In the downward thrust the leg is straight and the foot may or may not be extended. The six-beat kick is the most popular.

As in the free style, the muscles of the chest, back, shoulders, and arms furnish the power for the back crawl. In the catch and pull phases the arm power comes from the shoulder flexors and adductors (latissimus dorsi, pectoralis major, anterior deltoid). Otherwise the muscular action is very similar to that of the free style and the same muscles are in need of strength development.

Breast Stroke

Although it is the slowest of the speed strokes, the breast stroke was the first stroke taught to beginners until recent years. There are three basic phases; the arm stroke, the kick, and breathing. The basic position is prone in the water with the back slightly arched and the head up and looking straight ahead. The position is not significantly different from that of the crawl stroke.

1. The arm stroke

The arm stroke is less powerful than in any of the other competitive strokes. At the beginning of the pull the arms should extend directly in front of the face with the palms of the hands down and about 4 inches below the water

As the pull begins, the hands swing out, back, and away from the body. There is a slightly downward movement in order to lift the head and shoulders for breathing purposes. The arms reach a depth of 12 to 16 inches in the pull. The elbows remain higher than the hands throughout the pull. When the arms have swept through a half-circle so that the hands are even with the shoulders, the recovery is begun. The hands are brought in to the body before thrusting them forward. At the beginning of the thrust the hands are about a foot apart, but meet as they extend over the head in a straight-arm position.

2. The leg kick

At the completion of the kick, the legs should be straight, the feet together, and the toes pointed. The recovery begins with a flexing of the knees and hips. The knees are slightly apart and the feet are together during the first part of the recovery. The heels are drawn as closely as possible to the hips as the knees spread laterally apart. At the same time the feet are flexed so that the toes are closer to the shins. In the thrust the legs come further apart and a whiplike motion begins. The feet and the knees go outward and perform a circle which is completed when the legs come together. When the legs are at their farthest point apart the toes are slightly out. The knees lead the movement back together with the ankles trailing only slightly behind. When the feet are about a foot apart the feet are rotated in and extended downward. The swimmer should feel a thrust, a whip out and in, in a circular motion, and a squeeze as the legs close. Pressure should be felt from the knees down through the feet.

3. Coordination and breathing

The arms and legs alternate in their driving action, and there is a glide during the arm recovery. When the arms are pulling, the legs are cocking for the kick. At the end of the arm pull the legs are ready to whip together. The arms quickly begin their recovery as the legs squeeze together. The leg kick is rapid and is finished before the arms have completed the recovery. The arms thrust forward for the next arm pull and there is a short glide, because the legs are also extended. During the arm pull the head is out of the water so that air can be inhaled through the mouth. During the leg kick and the arm recovery the face is underwater and the air is exhaled. A breath is usually taken on every other stroke in the longer races and as seldom as possible in the short sprints.

Although the breast stroke bears little similarity to the free style, the arm and shoulder muscles that power the stroke are the same. The shoulder adductors (latissimus dorsi, pectoralis major), the forearm flexors (biceps, brachialis), extensors (triceps) and pronators (pronator teres and quadratus), and the wrist and hand flexors (flexor carpi group) are those that need extra developmemt. The leg kick is performed with a powerful adduction (adductors) at the hips and an inward rotation (tibialis posterior) and extension of the feet (soleus, gastrocnemius). Because the leg kick plays a much more prominent part a the breast stroke than it does in the free style, it is very important that the leg uscles be well strengthened for the breast stroker.

Butterfly Stroke

Since its development at the University of Iowa in 1934, the butterfly stroke with the dolphin kick has been used reluctantly. The stroke is an outgrowth of the breast stroke and because it defied tradition and is more strenuous than the conventional stroke it has gone through a long period of criticism before gaining recognition and legality in recent years. Today it is one of the fastest racing strokes because of the rapid above-water arms recovery in the butterfly action, and the utilization of the powerful leg thrust in the dolphin fishtail action.

The butterfly is an arm stroke fundamentally similar to that of the free-style stroke, the only difference being that both arms and legs move together in unison. In the free style, the same actions of both arms and legs are executed in alternating movements. The stroke is dominated by the kick, which resembles the tail movement of a flat-tailed dolphin.

1.   The arm stroke

The arms enter the water simultaneously, extending straight ahead. The wrists are partially flexed and the hands are about 8 to 10 inches apart with the palms turned outward. In the catch the shoulders are drawn over the arms by the force of the water against the hands as the arms extend. The pull is the same as in the free style, the elbows remaining slightly flexed. The hands push against the water to a point approximately even with the hips before thay are lifted out and the recovery is made in a low sweeping movement above the water. In this movement the arms are as relaxed as possible and carried with the elbows and little fingers up. As they pass the shoulders they are slightly rotated so that the hands face the water as they are pressed in, with as little splash but as quickly as possible.

2.   The leg stroke

The dolphin kick is similar to that of the flutter kick in the free style, except that both legs kick in unison. On the downward stroke the knees are somewhat flexed until almost the end of the beat. At this point the knees straighten powerfully, exerting a whip-like action on the feet as the latter flex slightly. On the upstroke the legs are straight until they reach the midline of the body. The knees begin bending and the feet extending at this point. As the legs weave up and down they press backward against the water, propelling the body forward.

3. Breathing and Coordination

Air is inhaled when the arms are about halfway through the recovery and during the downstroke of the kick. There are usually two leg strokes to one arm stroke. To maintain this ratio the swimmer must pull the arms through and recover very quickly in order to keep up with the leg action.

The muscular action of the dolphin butterfly stroke is almost identical t that of the free style. The very same muscles are involved, but they work ir different coordinated movement. In performing exercises to strengthen the muscles for the dolphin butterfly it is relatively simple to employ barbell exercises that will closely simulate the action of this stroke. However, in the crawl stroke the right and left sides of the body alternate actions and the exercise routines are more complicated. Both strokes are extremely vigorous and require excellent physical strength in the same muscle groups.

SUPPLEMENTARY EXERCISES AND DRILLS

Supplementary exercises are described primarily for joint flexibility and body conditioning. Joint flexibility is probably more important for a competitive swimmer than for any other athlete. Restricted joint movement not only prevents the full stroke movement necessary for maximum speed and power, but usually is accompanied by a poorly coordinated stroke. Poor flexibility can result from an overdevelopment of one muscle group and an underdevelopment of the opposite (antagonist) group; or the cause may be that the daily physical habits of an individual don't require a full range of movement in certain joints, and the muscles surrounding these joints gradually shorten as they adapt to their environment. In either event there are two good methods to assure full range of motion in a joint:

1. Developing equally the muscles on each side of the joint
2. Practicing stretching exercises with the muscles on each side of the joint

In a well-planned weight-training program there are exercises for each major muscle group, and opposite muscles are equally developed. It is also extremely important that each exercise be carried through a full range of motion. To further assure joint flexibility, a swimmer should spend a few minutes each day stretching the muscles on each side of the most important joints. Some of the better stretching exercises are included in this chapter. Many more are available in specialized swimming books listed in the references at the end of the chapter. The program of stretching exercises should be varied occasionally by substituting new exercises and changing the exercise order. They should be done after a brief warm-up and before the weight-training or swimming program.

The conditioning drills described below are designed to improve a swimmer's muscular strength and endurance. Although a general weight-training program plus some cross-country running may suffice, there are some specialized exercises not usually included in the regular routines that swimmers should use for spot development of specific swimming muscles. The training program hould be as closely associated with swimming activities as possible, and vimming drills should be a regular part of any training program for competitive 'mmers.

Flexibility drills

81.   Neck stretching

Stand with the body erect and head up. One the count of "one," touch the chin as far down on the chest as possible, stretching the muscles in the back of the neck. On "two," tilt the head back as far as possible, stretching the muscles on the front of the neck. On "three," touch the chin to the point of the right shoulder without lifting the shoulder, and on "four," touch the chin to the left shoulder. On "five," circumduct the head completely around the neck, stretching the neck muscles as much as possible.

82.   Shoulder stretching

Grasp an overhead bar, using the overhand grip with the hands close together. The body should hang so that the feet are free of the floor. Hang in a completely relaxed position as long as it is comfortable. This may be only a few seconds. Perform the same exercise using the underhand grip. The shoulders can also be stretched using the Dumbbell Circle (51) or similar exercises.

83.   Chest stretching

Two chairs or benches are placed beside each other, slightly farther apart than the width of the shoulders. Place a hand on each bench and extend the arms and legs in a push-up position. The toes are pointed so that the leg weight rests on the insteps or tops of the feet. Keep the head up and slowly lower the body between the benches so that the chest is well below the top of the benches; then push up to the starting position. The exercise may be varied by placing the feet on a third chair.

84.   Chest stretching

Swimmers work in pairs to perform this exercise. One swimmer sits on the floor with his arms held out. The partner stands behind him and grasps the arms at the elbows, placing one knee between the shoulder blades. The partner slowly pulls on the elbows and carries them up and down in a circular motion, stretching the muscles of the chest and shoulders.

85.   Low back and hamstring stretching

Start in the squat position, grasping under the front of the shoes with the fingers. Straighten the knees, keeping the feet flat on the floor and maintaining the grasp on the shoes. Return to the starting position and repeat. This exercise may also be done by lying on the back and grasping the toes in the same manner.

86.   Low back and hamstring stretching

Sit on the floor with the legs spread wide. Place the left hand on the left ankle and the right hand on the inside of the left thigh. Relax the low back muscles and pull the body down so the head touches the left leg. Return to the starting position and pull the body down to the right leg in the same manner. Keep the toes pointed and the legs straight so that the hamstrings will also be fully stretched.

87.   Low back and hamstring stretching

Start by lying flat on the back with the shoulders and elbows contacting the floor. Keeping the right leg perfectly straight, raise it to a perpendicular position and swing it across the body until the foot touches the floor on the opposite side. Repeat with the left leg.

88.   Hip stretching

Start in a striding position with the left leg forward. Lower the hips so that the left leg is bent, with the knee ahead of the ankle, and the right leg is extended behind. Lean forward at the waist and balance with the hands, maintaining most of the weight on the front leg. Bob the hips up and down, keeping the right leg extended behind. Change the positions of the legs and repeat.

89.   Quadricep stretching

Stand erect and flex the right leg at the hip and knee, grasping the foot with the right hand. Pull on the foot, carefully exerting a stretch on the quadricep muscles. Change the positions of the legs and repeat with the left leg.

90.   Ankle stretching

Stand facing a wall with the arms reaching out so that the fingertips barely touch. Lean toward the wall, keeping the body straight and the feet flat on the floor. Catch the body with the arms extended. Bend the arms so that the body goes closer to the wall, stretching the Achilles tendon.

91.   Ankle stretching

Kneel with the feet extended so that the body weight is supported on the knees and the insteps of the feet. Sit back on the heels, placing the hands on the floor at the sides to support some of the weight. Bend backward and rock the weight on the insteps.

The abdominal flexors can also be stretched in this exercise by bending backwards until the back of the head touches the floor. Return to the starting position, using the arms to assist if necessary.

92.   Ankle stretching

Sit on the floor and bend the knees so that the feet can be comfortably reached. Reach and grasp the left foot, the ball of the foot with the left hand and the ankle with the right. Manipulate the foot in a full range of motion with the left hand, stretching the joint in each position. Finish by extending the leg and pulling on the ball of the foot with both hands in order to stretch the Achilles tendon. Change foot positions and repeat.

General Conditioning Drills

93.   Back extension

One swimmer lies face down on the edge of a table so that the hips come directly over the edge and the upper trunk extends beyond. A teammate places his hands over the swimmer's legs to anchor him to the table. The first swimmer holds his hands behind his head and slowly raises the head and shoulders as high as possible; then lowers them as far as possible. Vary the exercise by twisting to the right on one repetition, then to the left on the next.

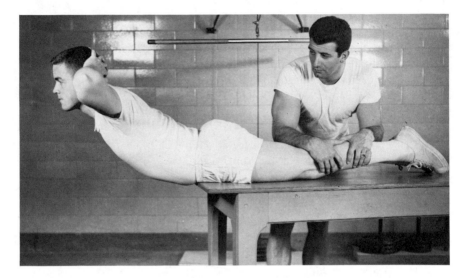

Figure 70. Back Extension

94. Latissimus dorsi machine

Grasp the handle of the "Lat" machine with the hands in the same relative position as in an actual swimming stroke (free style or butterfly). Position the body and set the machine so that the handle can be pulled down in the same movement as in the actual stroke. Increase the weight loads as in the other weight-training exercises, maintaining good form in each repetition.

95. Supine butterfly

Lie face up on the bench, holding a pair of dumbbells in an arm-extended position above the chest. In a motion simulating the butterfly stroke, describe a circular movement with each dumbbell, returning to the starting position. This exercise may be varied by simulating the free style or back crawl movements.

96. Pull

A conditioning drill used almost universally with good success is to bind the feet together and swim the desired stroke using the arms only. This drill should be practiced for arm endurance during the pre-season conditioning program, and many coaches continue to use it throughout the season.

97. Kick

Hold a kickboard at arms length in front of the body. Push off and in a prone position, with the head under water, practice the desired leg kick. Some

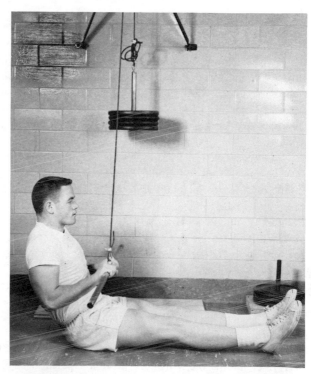

Figure 71. Latissimus
Dorsi Machine

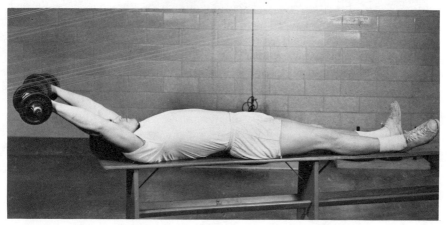

Figure 72. Supine Butterfly

coaches prefer not to use the kickboard because the swimmers are tempted to hold their heads too high in quest of air. Instead they either have the swimmer extend his hands out front with no support or hold them down by the sides.

OFF-SEASON PROGRAM

The off-season training program incorporates the use of the barbell only. In this way a complete squad can train as a unit with a minimum amount of lost time from weight changes. If a swimmer is training alone and time isn't a factor there are several dumbbell exercises that should prove very beneficial. The Lateral Raise, Supine (24) and the Supine Butterfly (95), are two exercises that should be added to the program. Alternate dumbbell presses and pullovers are also good.

Other barbell exercises may be selected to supplement the program. They may be substituted for similar exercises in the regular program or may be added to the program on planned variety days. Some of the more valuable additional exercises are Rowing (12), Neck Isometric Exercises (8, 9) and work with the Latissimus Dorsi Machine (94). If a "Lat" machine is available it should be included in the basic program to be used each training day. On the variety days perform only the first set of all the basic exercises so that the others may be added without lengthening the workout.

The flexibility drills should be practiced in the order listed as a part of the warm-up before each training session. These exercises should be used with caution because there is danger of pulling a muscle if it isn't properly readied for stretching. Jogging and alternate toe-touches should first be performed to stimulate circulation and warm up the muscles. The exercises should then be performed in the order listed. The first repetition of each exercise should be a cautious one, thereafter applying greater stretch on the muscles with each additional execution. If there is restricted movement in the joints it helps to bounce gently in order to put additional stretch on the surrounding muscles.

With only a few exceptions the lifting program is the same for all swimmers. Straight-arm pullovers should be performed by cheating slightly in order to closely simulate the actual butterfly or free style motion. Back strokers should perform additional work on the hand and shoulder flexors by adding a wrist curl and a stiff-armed curl, and breast strokers should add leg adductor exercises with the iron shoe and extra quadricep exercises. Otherwise the suggested program should be sufficient for specialists in all four strokes.

The off-season program should be practiced in the spring and in the summer. It can be practiced in the fall, but there are only a couple of months available between the opening of school and the time for hard training in the pool. If the fall season is selected, the alternate-day program should be changed so that the swimming program is much more vigorous than the one suggested.

Lifting Program

Exercise	Repetitions	Sets
Flexibility Drills		
1. Jogging (running in place if raining)	1 lap or 1 minute	1
2. Alternate toe touches	10	1

Lifting Program (cont.)

Exercise	Repetitions	Sets
Flexibility Drills		
3. Neck stretching (81)	3 each direction	1
4. Dumbbell circle (51)	5 each direction	1
5. Chest stretching (83)	3 to 5	1
6. Low back and hamstring stretching (86)	3 to 5	1
7. Hip stretching (88)	3 to 5	1
8. Quadricep stretching (89)	3 to 5	1
9. Ankle stretching (90)	3 to 5	1
10. Ankle stretching (91)	3 to 5	1
Power Exercises		
1. Dumbbell swing (5)	10	1
2. Squat jump (1)	15	1
3. Modified clean (2)	10	1
4. Power press (4)	10	1
Basic Exercises		
1. Squat (28)	15-maximum	2
2. Bench press (22)	10-maximum	2
3. Sit-up (26)	25-maximum to 100	2
4. Overhead press (11)	10-maximum	2
5. Two-arm curl (16)	10-maximum	2
6. Back extension (93)	10-maximum	2
7. Rowing upright (13)	10-maximum	2
8. Straight-arm pullover (23)	10-maximum	2
9. Chinning (overhand) (18)	maximum	1

Power Rack Program (Hold each exercise approximately seven seconds)

1. Heel-raise (38)
2. Overhead press (34)
3. Curl (33)
4. Tricep (17)
5. Upright rowing (35)
6. Dead lift (36)

Alternate-day Program

During the off-season; some coaches prefer that their swimmers stay away
ı the swimming pool. Records continue to be broken each year, however, by

swimmers who train the year round. On alternate days of the off-season weight-training program, some swimming should be done so that the strength and flexibility derived from the program can be associated with the movement patterns of the swimming strokes. During this time the concentration should be on form, technique, relaxation and breathing.

The suggested program should be used only as a point of departure and should be adjusted to fit individual capabilities. It is intended as a very mild program. For beginning swimmers it may be too vigorous; for the more advanced it may be too mild. The beginner should complete the entire workout within 30 to 40 minutes, whereas the advanced competitor should work at least 90 minutes.

Alternate-day program

Exercise	Repetitions	Sets
Flexibility Drills		
1. Dumbbell circle (51)	5 each direction	1
2. Chest stretching (83)	3 to 5	1
3. Low back and hamstring stretching (86)	3 to 5	1
4. Ankle stretching (90)	3 to 5	1

Conditioning Drills

1. Swim 400 yards
   100 yards butterfly
   100 yards free style
   100 yards back crawl
   100 yards breaststroke
2. Swim 200 yards best stroke
3. Kick (97) 100 yards
4. Pull (96) 100 yards
5. Swim 10 sprints (25 yards)

Power Rack Program (Hold each exercise approximately seven seconds)

1. Heel-raise (38)
2. Overhead press (34)
3. Curl (33)
4. Tricep (17)
5. Upright rowing (35)
6. Dead lift (36)

PRE-SEASON PROGRAM

During the six weeks before official practice begins, the time devoted to weight training should be lessened and a larger percentage of the swimmers' practice should be in the water. The off-season lifting program should be followed for the first three weeks with only a few modifications. The same flexibility exercises should be performed as listed. However, the power exercises should be omitted and the basic exercise program should be restricted to one set of each exercise, except for the Squat (28) Straight-Arm Pullover (23) Back Extension (93), and Sit-up (26). These exercises should continue to be performed for three sets.

The warm-up should be in the form of swimming drills in which form, relaxation, and breathing are still of primary importance. Occasional sprint work should be practiced. These drills should be performed *before* the weight-training program so that the muscles will not be too tired to execute them properly.

During the second three weeks the swimming drills are gradually increased and the amount of time devoted to lifting is gradually decreased. Only one set of the weight-training exercises are performed. Although the program charts show this to be a sharp change at the end of three weeks, in reality the change of emphasis from weight training to swimming should be a gradual process. Especially should the increase in swimming be gradually effected.

During the second three weeks the alternate-day program should occasionally be spiced with various races and relays in order to add variety to the program.

Jogging should be a part of the entire pre-season program so that improved endurance can gradually be achieved.

Training Program, First Three Weeks

Lifting program

Exercise	Repetitions	Sets
Warm-up		
1. Swim 200 yards		
50 yards butterfly		
50 yards free style		
50 yards back crawl		
50 yards breaststroke		
2. Pull (96) 150 yards best stroke		
3. Kick (97) 150 yards best stroke		
4. Swim 400 yards best stroke		

Training Program, First Three Weeks

Lifting program (cont.)

Exercise	Repetitions	Sets
Flexibility Drills		
Same as off-season program		
Basic Exercises		
1. Squat (28)	15-maximum	2
2. Bench press (22)	10-maximum	2
3. Sit-up (26)	50	1
4. Overhead press (11)	10-maximum	2
5. Two-arm curl (16)	10-maximum	2
6. Back extension (93)	maximum	1
7. Rowing upright (13)	10-maximum	2
8. Straight-arm pullover (23)	10-maximum	2
9. Chinning (overhand) (18)	maximum	1
Endurance Exercise		
1. Jogging (indoors)	half-mile	1

Alternate-day program

Exercise	Repetitions	Sets
Flexibility Drills		
Same as off-season program		
Endurance Exercise		
1. Jogging	one mile	
Conditioning Exercises		
1. Swim 400 yards		
100 yards butterfly		
100 yards free style		
100 yards back crawl		
100 yards breaststroke		
2. Pull (96) 200 yards best stroke		
3. Kick (97) 200 yards best stroke		
4. Swim 200 yards best stroke		
5. Swim 10 sprints (25 yards)		
6. Swim 400 yards (up slow, back fast)		

Training Program, First Three Weeks

Alternate-day program (cont.)

Exercise	Repetitions	Sets

Power Rack Program (Hold each exercise approximately seven seconds)

1. Heel-raise (38)
2. Overhead press (34)
3. Curl (33)
4. Tricep (17)
5. Upright rowing (35)
6. Dead lift (36)

Training Program, Last Three Weeks

Lifting program

Exercise	Repetitions	Sets

Flexibility Drills

Same as off-season program

Warm-up

1. Swim 400 yards
   100 yards butterfly
   100 yards free style
   100 yards back crawl
   100 yards breaststroke
2. Pull (96) 200 yards best stroke
3. Kick (97) 200 yards best stroke
4. Swim 500 yards best stroke

Basic Exercises

Exercise	Repetitions	Sets
1. Squat (28)	maximum	1
2. Bench press (22)	maximum	1
3. Sit-up (26)	50	1
4. Overhead press (11)	maximum	1
5. Two-arm curl (16)	maximum	1
6. Back extension (93)	maximum	1
7. Rowing upright (13)	10	1
8. Straight-arm pullover (23)	maximum	1
9. Chinning (overhand) (18)	maximum	

Training Program, Last Three Weeks

Lifting program (cont.)

Exercise	Repetitions	Sets
Endurance Exercise		
1. Jogging (indoors)	one mile	1

Alternate-day program

Exercise	Repetitions	Sets
Flexibility Drills		
Same as off-season program		
Endurance Exercise		
1. Jogging	one mile	1

Conditioning Exercises

1. Swim 400 yards
   100 yards butterfly
   100 yards free style
   100 yards back crawl
   100 yards breaststroke
2. Pull (96) 300 yards best stroke
3. Kick (97) 300 yards best stroke
4. Swim 300 yards best stroke
5. Swim 20 sprints (25 yards)
6. Swim 400 yards (up slow, back fast)

Power Rack Program (Hold each exercise approximately seven seconds)

1. Heel-raise (38)
2. Overhead press (34)
3. Curl (33)
4. Tricep (17)
5. Upright rowing (35)
6. Dead lift (36)

IN-SEASON PROGRAM

During the competitive season one to two weight-training sessions a week are usually sufficient to maintain strength previously gained through a weight program. The best day to lift is usually the next day or two after a meet.

A program similar to one suggested for the last three weeks before official practice is recommended. If a boy is competing regularly this is usually as much lifting as he should attempt. However, if a swimmer is losing because he lacks basic body strength, a weight-training program should be a part of his workout on at least three days a week.

The flexibility drills should be a part of every practice day. On days that no lifting is being done the drills should be followed with sit-ups, back extensions, and push-ups before the water workout is started. These calisthenics in conjunction with the once-a-week lifting program will help maintain the muscles in a fine degree of condition.

If the entire program is designed to prepare the swimmers for an end of season event, heavy lifting should be continued at least three days a week until about ten days before the meet.

SELECTED REFERENCES

Armbruster, David A., Robert H. Allen, and Bruce Harlan, *Swimming and Diving*. St. Louis: The C. V. Mosby Company, 1958.

Barr, Alfred S., Ben F. Grady, and Lt. Commander John H. Higgins, *Swimming and Diving*. New York: A. S. Barnes & Company, 1950.

Counsilman, James E., *The Science of Swimming*. Englewood Cliffs, N.J.: Prentice-Hall, Inc., 1968.

Kiphuth, Robert J. H., *Swimming*. New York. A. S. Barnes & Company, 1942.

Mann, Matt, and Charles C. Fries, *Swimming, Fundamentals*. Englewood Cliffs, N.J.: Prentice-Hall, Inc., 1940.

10

WEIGHT TRAINING
IN TRACK AND FIELD

Weight training has completely revolutionized all track and field training methods. Until the 1960s, weight training was strictly taboo with most track men, but today it is extremely popular. The list of weight-trained track and field champions who pioneered the use of weights in track in the early sixties is endless. Prominent American stars were Rafer Johnson and Milton Campbell in the decathlon; Mal Whitfield in the middle distances; John Thomas in the high jump; Bob Richards, Don Bragg, and Bob Gutowski in the pole vault; Bill Nieder, Dallas Long, Dave Davis, and Parry O'Brien in the shot-put; Ray Norton and Dave Sime in the sprints; Fortune Gordien and Al Oerter in the discus; Bob Backus and Harold Connolly in the hammer throw, and Bud Held and Steve Seymour in the javelin. In recent years almost all of the U.S. track champions have used some form of weight training.

Foreign track and field stars are also using weight training with spectacular success. In Australia, England, and Russia the use of weights is reportedly a basic part of their training programs. As a result, the assault on world track and field records has been little short of fantastic. As weight training methods in track and field are improved and woven into the basic training routines, the present records will continue to fall.

Although the rise of weight training and the rash of broken track and field records follow somewhat parallel courses, it should be noted that many factors other than strength are necessary to break a record in any of the events. Speed, agility, flexibility, endurance, and skill are all important. The events must be practiced religiously to develop the necessary skill and to apply the speed, strength, flexibility, and endurance that might be derived from a weight-training program. A program that combines the practice of the athlete's event with a complete program of conditioning and training will yield the most satsifactory results. Such a program requires a tremendous amount of dedication and self-sacrifice if the desired results are to be accomplished.

Because many track and field events are so completely different, there is no single weight program or general training program that will suffice for all. More than in any other sport, training for track and field is an individual matter. Coaches should work out training programs for each team member and should supervise their programs as closely as possible. However, most coaches are overloaded with duties and cannot possibly supervise the workout of all squad members. Individual squad members must assume a great deal of personal responsibility in carrying out their program.

The weight-training programs, or modifications, should be practiced at least eight to ten months a year. They should usually be done three days a week, and regularly supplemented with a wide variety of other exercises. Naturally, the programs should be modified during the season so that the athlete can perform at his best in his specialty. A good procedure is to practice a variety of exercises with lighter weights than usual two days before a meet, and then not lift on the day preceding and the day of the meet. As in other sports, if the lifting program is practiced during the season, the track practice session should be finished before the weight-training program is started.

It is important to keep in mind the ultimate objective of the training program. If the trainee is working toward a championship meet for a peak performance, it might very well be that he should continue a fairly heavy lifting program during the competitive season, with little or no modification. If the regular schedule is more important, the lifting program should be modified. Because participation in track and field is virtually a year-round activity, there isn't really an off-season. For that reason off-season, pre-season, and in-season workouts are not included in this chapter. It is left to the judgement of the participant with the suggestion that some form of weight training be continued throughout with special emphasis being placed on heavy strength-building if there is an off-season, but centering most of the training around power development immediately prior to and during the actual season.

Most track and field events are highly specialized, and it is very unusual for an athlete to excel in more than one or two events. Running, hurdling, and jumping are the most closely related skills and involve almost identical muscular actions. Leg speed and power are the two most fundamental requirements, and individuals who are blessed with these qualities may train for any one of the three skills and attain some degree of success. Because these skills are so closely related and involve virtually the same muscle groups, only one weight-training program is presented for all three. However, the general conditioning programs are quite different for these events, and will necessitate a variety of training techniques.

The shot-put, javelin throw, and the discus throw are entirely different and require a different type of athlete. Success in these weight events and the pole vault requires much greater arm and shoulder power than in the running and jumping events. As a matter of fact, exceptional strength is more important to the weight men than to almost any other athlete. The pole vaulter has to be proportionately as powerful as any athlete. He is usually much smaller than the weight men, but he must have tremendous power to completely control his body weight. In each of these skills the techniques, and subsequently the muscular actions, are quite different. Each can be improved through weight training, but because of their dissimilarity of actions the training program for each is quite different. Therefore, the techniques and muscular actions are described separately and a slightly different weight-training program is suggested for each skill.

SUPPLEMENTARY EXERCISES

Joint flexibility is extremely important to all track and field men and they need to undergo a routine of exercises each day to improve the range of movement in the joints. The hurdlers and high jumpers especially need these exercises, probably as much as twenty minutes a day before they begin their organized practice session.

There is a great need for caution in performing stretching exercises or they can do more harm than good. Go easy at first and warm-up properly before attempting them. Increase the degree of stretch on the muscles by gently bobbing as the stretch is applied, not by pulling and tugging. The exercises should be done after some jogging and before the sprints. In order to be certain enough warm-up activity is provided they should be performed in the order listed. The side-straddle hop and the squat thrust should be done at least fifteen times.

Sprints should be run after the flexibility exercises. In order to guard against pulled muscles, it is a good plan to start the first few sprints with an easy stride, build up quickly to a hard sprint, and then ease off to a short jog before stopping.

Flexibility Drills

98. Side-straddle hop
Stand erect with hands at the sides. Jump into the air bringing the arms in a wide arc to an overhead position and the legs out to a straddle position. Return to the starting position by jumping again, bringing the arms in the same arc to the original position and the legs back together. This is one of the better warm-up drills.

99.   Squat thrust

For this warm-up drill stand erect with the hands at the sides. On a count of "one" squat to the floor, putting the hands on the floor between the knees. On "two" thrust the legs out behind in a push-up position. Bring them back to the squat position on "three," and stand erect on "four." This drill is often changed to six counts by inserting a push-up on counts "three" and "four."

100.   Crossover

This is an excellent exercise to stretch the lower back and hamstring muscles. Stand erect with the legs crossed. Keeping the legs straight, reach down and across and touch beside the right foot with the right hand on the count of "one." Stand erect on "two." Touch beside the left foot with the left hand on "three," and stand erect on "four."

101.   Knee hug

A good drill for simultaneously stretching the knee flexor and hip extensor muscles is the Knee Hug. Stand erect and grasp one leg at the shin and pull it up so that the knee comes as high as possible. Repeat with the other leg.

102.   Hurdle stretch

Take a position beside the hurdle and place the right leg on the top, in the hurdling position. Touch the toes of the left foot with both hands. Come to an erect position with the head back, holding the hurdle with the right hand. Turn around and perform the same exercise with the left leg on the hurdle. This exercise stretches the adductor muscles of the leg along with the extensors of the back.

103.   Leg and crotch extension

This is a good exercise to stretch the hip and knee flexors and extensors. Stand with one foot on the ground and hook the heel of the other foot over the hurdle. Hold the hurdle with both hands and bob up and down. Repeat with the other foot on the hurdle.

104.   Hurdle stretch on ground

Sit on the ground and take the hurdle position. Hold the front leg with the hands and touch the head to the knee. Rock back to a full back extension and repeat, maintaining the hurdle position. This drill, like the Hurdle Stretch, helps stretch the leg adductors and lower back flexor muscles.

DISCUSSION OF RUNNING, HURDLING, AND JUMPING SKILLS

Running

The most important part of any dash is the start, because a good percentage of races is decided in the first five strides. As the distance of the race increases the importance of the start decreases, so that in the longer races it is merely a maneuver for running position.

The better sprinters develop good starts by experimenting with foot spacing until they find a starting position suitable to them. When proper foot spacing has been determined, the runner measures the distance from the starting line to each of the starting blocks. The right-footed sprinter should place his right foot on the front block and his left foot on the rear block.

In the "get set" position, the arms extend straight down from the shoulders with the wrists and hands chest-width apart. The weight is evenly distributed between the front foot and the finger tips. The hips are raised so that they are slightly higher than the shoulders. However, the head should not be raised because it tends to cause excessive tenseness in the neck and shoulders. The trunk, hips, legs and ankles are well-flexed as they coil for the start.

In the burst from the starting block the stronger push is from the right leg. while the left is used for a quick first step. The emphasis is not on a vigorous push against the rear block, but a continued drive from the front block. The rear. leg comes forward rapidly with the foot barely clearing the ground. The step should be a fairly long one, although not so long as to check forward momentum, and certainly not so short as to make balance difficult to maintain. During the first few strides the weight is mostly on the balls of the feet. Thereafter in the dashes, the heels drop down somewhat but don't usually touch the ground.

As the left foot drives through, the right arm is swung forward in the direction of the run. The left arm is swung forward as the right leg drives, and vigorous arm action is continued alternately with the leg drive.

During the first 15 yards of the race, the trunk gradually is raised to the normal sprinting position, with high knee action, long stride, and some forward lean. The back kick is at a minimum and arm action is relaxed and in, the arms not swinging across the midline of the body. The feet point straight ahead throughout the race.

In the longer races the form is essentially the same, except that the stride is not quite as long, the body lean is slightly less, the arm action is more in front of the body and less exaggerated, and the running is more rhythmical, relaxed, and less vigorous.

The most important muscles in running are obviously those of the legs and trunk. The legs furnish much of the actual driving force, but the trunk flexors and extensors stabilize the pelvis and provide strong support for the driving action of the legs. The extensors of the left hip (gluteus maximus, hamstrings), knee (quadriceps), and ankle (gastrocnemius, soleus) contract quickly to drive that leg from the starting block. The final impetus of the left foot is given by the flexors of the toes. The flexors of the left hip (iliopsoas) and knee (hamstrings) accomplish the first part of the high knee action as the leg swings forward. The leg actually starts back just before the ball of the foot contacts the ground, so that the body is almost over it at contact. The other gluteal muscles and the tensor fasciae latae contract to stabilize the pelvis.

The action of the right leg is almost identical. However, because it is flexed more at the joints, the muscles are able to contract over a greater range of motion and actually furnish a great deal more power in the first step than the left. The momentum provided by the action of the left leg helps make this possible.

The arms are alternately driven forward by the shoulder flexors (anterior deltoid, pectoralis major). The elbows remain flexed (bicips, brachialis) at approximately 90 degrees throughout the sprint.

The rib cage is elevated (intercostals) to provide for maximum breathing efficiency, and the neck is maintained in a slightly extended position (splenius capitis, semispinalis capitis) in spite of the forward lean of the body. In the longer races there is less body lean, and therefore, little reason for strong contraction of the neck extensors.

Hurdling

In running the hurdles, the start and the dash between each hurdle are identical to the sprints. The hurdler must take great care in the first few steps to bring the take-off foot to the correct distance from the hurdles and must practice to correct a faulty stride between the hurdles. The proper technique in clearing the hurdle is accomplished with much hard work and good instruction. For a good sprinter, the mastery of the hurdles is largely a matter of courage and the ability to master the hurdling form. Otherwise, the dash is the same and the same powerful leg muscles are responsible for success. With only one exception, the hurdler should train with the sprinter. Running the hurdles demands that the hip and knee joints have an exceptionally good range of motion. Leg flexibility exercises are extremely valuable for these boys and should be a part of each workout. Otherwise the weight-training program should be identical to that of the sprinter.

Jumping

The broad jumper must be the same type of athlete as the sprinter and must have basically the same muscular development. Therefore, his weight program should be almost identical. There is, however, a greater difference in the skill of the high jumper. Where the runners and broad jumpers must aim to project their body forward with a maximum force, the high jumper must concentrate all of his efforts in jumping straight up.

The high jumper approaches the bar from an angle. Some of the best jumpers take only three short steps and four long strides before the takeoff. Others have enjoyed outstanding success by running hard all the way to the takeoff. Regardless of the speed of the approach, the left heel is planted hard or the last stride. With the hard heel-plant, all forward momentum is stopped and the drive is straight up from the toes. The right leg swings straight up and over the bar. The left leg trails so that the legs straddle the bar as the body goes over.

The force for the jump is generated by the same muscles involved in running, although the immediate objectives are different. The plantar flexors of the left foot (gastrocnemius, soleus), the knee extensors (quadriceps), and the hip extensors (gluteus maximus) of the left leg and the thigh flexors (iliopsoas) of the right leg are most important; but their antagonistic muscles must be equally developed to maintain balance. Therefore, the same program is recommended as for the runners and broad jumpers, plus additional time devoted to flexibility drills.

Weight-training Program

The weight program for runners, jumpers, and hurdlers is basic to all track programs. The exercises are mostly basic and the program is complete enough to enable any track and field man to profit from it. The programs for all of the other track and field events listed in this book are based on this basic program.

Lifting program

Exercise	Repetitions	Sets
Warm-up		
1. Jogging	half-mile	1
2. Flexibility exercises (98 thru 104)		
3. Sprints	5	1
Power Exercises		
1. Modified clean (2)	10	1
2. Power press (4)	10	1
3. Squat jump (1)	15	1
4. Power curl (3)	10	1
Basic Exercises		
1. Squat (28)	15-maximum	2
2. Heel-raise (30)	15-maximum	2
3. Sit-up (26)	25-maximum to 100	2
4. Bench press (22)	10-maximum	2
5. Dead lift, Straight legs (25)	10-10-10	3
6. Overhead press (11)	10-maximum	2
7. Two-arm curl (16)	10-maximum	2

Lifting program (cont.)

Exercise	Repetitions	Sets
8. Rowing upright (13)	10-maximum	2
9. Straight-arm pullover (23)	10-maximum	2

Power Rack Program (Hold each exercise approximately seven seconds)
1. Heel-raise (38)
2. Overhead press (34)
3. Curl (33)
4. Tricep (17)
5. Upright rowing (35)
6. Dead lift (36)

DISCUSSION OF DISCUS THROWING

The discus is held in the throwing hand with the fingers spread wide and the first joint gripping the edge. The thumb is flat against the side of the discus and extends in a line with the forearms. There are several modifications of the grip, depending mostly on the size of the hand.

The stance and the preliminary movements are important and should not be regarded lightly. The thrower usually stands with his feet parallel and faces the back of the circle. The discus may be swung backward and slightly downward several times in preparation for the throw. In the last swing the head and shoulders turn as they cock with the swing and most of the weight is borne on the right leg (right-handed thrower). The left leg and arm help to maintain balance.

As the discus reaches the back of the last swing, the left leg steps forward slightly and the first pivot is made on the left foot. The body falls in the direction of the throw and pivots speedily, first on the left foot, then on the right. The right arm is fully extended and drags behind the shoulder, the hand carrying the discus at approximately hip level. The left arm is partially flexed and continues to aid in balance.

As the body rotates it should be kept fairly low, with the knees bent slightly and the weight on the balls of the feet. As the thrower completes the pivot with the right foot he should be facing the front of the circle, the left leg planted firmly near the front of the circle, and the body weight gathered over the right leg. Immediately the right leg is extended powerfully and the weight is shifted to the left side. The hips and shoulders rotate to the left followed by the whip-like action of the throwing arm. The discus is released at about shoulder level with a clockwise spin off the index finger at approximately a 30-degree angle.

The recovery is made by bringing the right leg around and planting the right foot a few inches from the edge of the circle and drawing the left arm and leg backward to assist in balancing.

The cocking action is brought about by the horizontal extensors of the right shoulder (posterior deltoid, teres minor), the extensors of the right elbow (triceps), the extensors of the left knee (quadriceps) and ankle (gastrocnemius, soleus), and the rotators of the trunk (obliques, quadratus lumborum).

The twisting of the body to the left, as momentum is built up in preparation for the release, is accomplished primarily by the opposite trunk muscles plus the extensors of the legs. The movements are very fast, allowing the throwing arm to drag behind. As the left leg is planted firmly for the throw, there is a powerful extension of the right leg (gastrocnemius, soleus, quadriceps, gluteus maximus) and a twisting of the trunk to the left. The left arm is usually held away from the body and flexed for balance. The right arm is brought powerfully into action by the horizontal flexors of the shoulder (pectoralis major, anterior deltoid). The forearm is held pronated (pronator teres and pronator quadratus) and adducted until the last instant, when the wrist snaps through and imparts the final impetus. This is accomplished by the combined efforts of the flexor and extensor carpi muscles on the lateral (thumb) side of the hand.

Probably the most important muscles in performing the throw are the horizontal flexors of the shoulder. They impart a great deal of the power for the throw. Otherwise the entire body must be well-muscled and coordinated in order to generate a maximum amount of power, and to expend it in the right direction and manner at precisely the right time. The discus throw is a complex activity that requires many hours of practice before it can be done correctly.

Weight-training Program

The discus-lifting program is different from the javelin and shot programs because the throwing motion is quite different. Extra work must be done on the horizontal flexors of the shoulder, and these muscles should be exercised in a motion that resembles the discus throw. The lateral raises on the inclined bench are an excellent exercise for this reason. The wrist abductor exercise is included to help strengthen the muscles that provide the final impetus, and throwing the weighted plates should be practiced from a standing position. All types of sprinting, hurdling and jumping should supplement the training program.

Lifting program

Exercise	Repetitions	Sets
Warm-up		
1. Jogging	half-mile	1
2. Flexibility exercises (98 thru 104)		
3. Sprints	5	1
Power Exercises		
1. Modified clean (2)	10	1
2. Power press (4)	10	1
3. Squat jump (1)	15	1
4. Power curl (3)	10	1
Basic Exercises		
1. Squat (28)	15-maximum	2
2. Heel-raise (30)	15-maximum	2
3. Sit-up (26)	25-maximum to 100	2
4. Weighted plate throw	5 each with 10- and 25-lb. plate	
5. Dead lift (29)	12-10	2
6. Overhead press (11)	10	1
7. Two-arm curl (16)	10-maximum	3
8. Lateral raise, supine (24)	10-maximum	2
9. Wrist curl (20)	10	1
10. Reverse wrist curl (21)	10	1

Power Rack Program (Hold each exercise approximately seven seconds)
1. Overhead press (34)
2. Curl (33)
3. Tricep (17)
4. Upright rowing (35)

Supplementary Exercises for Alternate Days
1. Rope: climbing, skipping
2. Special events: high jump, low hurdles, running and standing broad jump, sprint
3. Weights: chinning, shoulder dip, tricep, trunk twist, wrist roller, wall pulley exercises, lateral raise on incline board, incline press

DISCUSSION OF JAVELIN THROWING

The thrower grasps the javelin at the rear of the cord so that the middle finger holds the shaft with one-half of the finger on the cord and one-half on the shaft, the tip of the finger barely touching the thumb. The third and fourth fingers grip the cord securely and the index finger grasps the shaft rather loosely. The javelin rests on the palm of the hand and along the inner side of the wrist.

There are several methods of carrying the javelin and of footwork just prior to and during the throw. The Finnish style seems to be the most acceptable. The javelin is carried over the shoulder with the point slightly down. The approach run varies from 50 to 100 feet. The thrower starts slowly with a relaxed stride, the speed increasing until the final action begins. During the final action, top speed should be maintained until the left foot is finally planted for the throw.

In the Finnish Front Cross Step there are five steps involved. At step *one* the right foot is planted straight ahead. At step *two* the left foot is pointed to the right. Step *three* is a crossover step with the right foot so that it is also planted pointing to the right. Step *four* is a long stride, bringing the left foot in line with the direction of the throw. In step *five* the recovery is made as the right foot is planted to prevent fouling. Recently, many javelin throwers have used two consecutive crossover steps with the right leg.

The thrower lands in the throwing position in step four with the feet well spread, the weight slightly back on the right leg, the right knee bent, the left side facing the direction of the throw, the throwing arm extended fully to the rear with the shoulder dipped and the body cocked back at the waist. This coiling action must be accomplished in spite of the fact that the thrower is running almost at top speed.

As the left foot strikes the ground the shoulders rotate to the left and the chest is thrust forward and held high. The right leg is powerfully extended as the body drives hard against a straight and firm left leg. The firm left leg stops the forward momentum of the body, but accelerates the arm and shoulder speed. As the throwing motion starts, the right hand trails well behind the elbow as it passes the shoulder. The hand passes at about ear level, and the javelin is released in front of and slightly above the right shoulder at an angle of approximately 40 degrees. The delivery should be straight over-arm with a complete extension of the right arm, the trunk, and the legs.

The muscles primarily responsible for throwing the javelin are essentially the same as those used in throwing a baseball. The most important ones are the abductors of the shoulder girdle (serratus anterior), the horizontal flexors of the shoulder (anterior deltoid, pectoralis major), the extensor of the elbow (triceps), the pronators of the forearm (pronator quadratus, pronator teres), and the flexors of the wrist (flexor carpi group). The trunk muscles are important for body rotation and the leg muscles are valuable in providing the necessary speed build-up. The right leg extensors (gluteus maximus, quadriceps, gastrocnemius, soleus) provide the final leg push.

Weight-training Program

Throwing a javelin is very similar to throwing a baseball. A javelin is considerably heavier, however, and throwing distance, not accuracy, is most important to success. Superior strength in the arm and shoulder muscles is mandatory for the javelin throw, and every effort should be made to increase it to a maximum. It should be pointed out, however, that the javelin throw is an extremely difficult skill to master. The ability to time the steps properly and to generate all of the power to explode at precisely the the right instant comes only after many hours of practice. Additional strength will be relatively ineffective if the fundamentals of throwing are not properly performed.

Because the javelin must be thrown with an explosive action after a run at nearly top speed, every effort should be made to improve the explosive force the body can generate. This can be done best by encouraging the throwers to perform each exercise at top speed. Practicing the sprint starts, sprints, hurdles, and the broad jump and high jump will also help improve the explosive force of the javelin thrower. The sprint should be practiced each day along with relaxed running, developing the stride to such a degree that the full concentration of the thrower can be directed toward the actual throwing phase. On the days that weight training isn't practiced, the sprint work and the javelin practice should be done early in the practice period. A program of calisthenics should follow, including some of the supplementary exercises. On lifting days any practice throwing should be done after the warm-up suggested in the lifting program.

Lifting program

Exercises	Repetitions	Sets
Warm-up		
1. Jogging	half-mile	1
2. Flexibility exercises (98 thru 104)		
3. Sprints	5	1
Power Exercises		
1. Modified clean (2)	10	1
2. Power press (4)	10	1
3. Squat jump (1)	15	1
4. Dumbbell swing (5)	10	1

Lifting program (cont.)

Exercise	Repetitions	Sets
Basic Exercises		
1. Dead lift (29)	15-maximum	2
2. Sit-up (26)	25-maximum to 100	2
3. Bench press (22)	10-maximum	2
4. Dead lift, Straight legs (25)	10-10	2
5. Straight-arm pullover (23)	10-maximum	2
6. Overhead press (11)	10-maximum	2
7. Two-arm curl (16)	10-maximum	2
8. Tricep (17)	10-maximum	2
9. Wrist curl (20)	10-maximum	2

Power Rack Program (Hold each exercise approximately seven seconds)
1. Overhead press (34)
2. Curl (33)
3. Tricep (17)
4. Upright rowing (35)

Supplementary Exercises
1. Rope: climbing, skipping
2. Special events: broad and high jump, low hurdles, sprints
3. Weights: heel-raise, knee-bend and shoulder press, latissimus machine exercises, reverse curl, shoulder dip, squat, wall pulley exercise, weighted javelin throwing, wrist pronation, wrist roller

DISCUSSION OF SHOT-PUTTING

The shot is held well up in the fingers of the right hand. The three middle fingers are spread slightly and are positioned behind the shot, while the thumb and little finger provide lateral support. The putter stands erect at the rear of the circle with the shot cradled against the neck. The right foot is pointed to the rear of the circle, the right knee is bent slightly, and the back faces the intended direction of the put. To maintain consistency, the eyes are focused on a spot several yards behind the ring.

The action is started with a deep bend of the body over the bent right leg, the left leg and back assuming a position that is almost parallel to the ground. The glide is started with a vigorous kick of the left leg and a simultaneous push and low glide with the right leg to the middle of the circle. The right foot is planted heavily in the center of the circle, facing slightly backward with the center of gravity directly over the right leg. The left foot lands against the center of the toeboard, pointing slightly forward. The right shoulder and arm are still cocked, the trunk is rotated to the right and in a crouched position.

The put is an explosive burst of power brought about by a rotation of the hips and shoulders to the left, an extension of the right arm, a horizontal flexion of the right shoulder, and an extension of the right hip and knee. The final impetus is provided by a forceful push off the ball of the right foot and a forward snap of the right wrist and a push with the fingers. The hand should follow the direction of the throw, the palm turning down and out. During the put the left arm snaps quickly across the body to aid in the rotation movement and balance.

In the follow-through, the putter rises high on the ball of the left foot and extends the right arm and body toward the direction of the put. He stays in the circle by executing a reverse, or snappy exchange of the position of the feet.

Certainly no other track event carries with it such an obvious need for strength as does the shot-put. Even though the action is primarily a full body movement, the need for power is primarily in the muscles of the arms and shoulders. The legs are almost as important, however, and a proportional amount of time should be spent in developing them.

The action preliminary to the actual putting phase is designed to build up terrific momentum across the circle, at the same time maintaining a putting position that will enable the putter to start the action from as fully cocked a position as possible. This action enables him to develop the power needed for the put over as long a range of motion as possible.

As the final action begins, the hips are pivoted powerfully to the left by the trunk rotators (obliques, quadratus lumborum) and the extensors of the right hip (gluteus maximus), acting with the flexors of the left knee (hamstrings). The left arm is extended horizontally (posterior deltoid, infraspinatus, teres minor) across the body to assist in the trunk rotation. The muscles on the right side simultaneously furnish the power for the put. The right shoulder girdle abductor (serratus anterior) contracts very powerfully to pull the shoulder girdle forward as the horizontal flexors of the shoulder (pectoralis major, anterior deltoid) contract to pull the upper arm around. Unlike the javelin throw, the elbow trails the hand throughout, enabling the elbow extensor (triceps) to contract vigorously to extend the arm at the elbow. The flexion of the wrists and fingers is caused by a vigorous contraction of the flexor carpi muscle group, and the forearm pronation as the shot is leaving the hand is caused by the pronator quadratus. The power for the right leg action is provided by the hip extensors (gluteus maximus), the knee extensors (quadriceps), and the foot plantar flexors (soleus, gastrocnemius).

Weight-training Program

Strength is obviously the most important characteristic of good shot men; but as in most sports, strength alone is not enough. Speed and agility are extremely important, as evidenced by the fact that most of the leading putters practice sprinting; the Olympic champion, Bill Nieder, reportedly played handball regularly. Putting the shot requires excellent body control and balance. Therefore, only the better-coordinated athletes succeed at it.

The weight-training program is designed with a heavy concentration of exercises that develop the anterior deltoid, serratus anterior, pectoralis major, and tricep muscles — all of which are important to the actual putting motion. Other exercises are also included to insure general body development and strengthening of antagonistic muscles.

Of the supplementary exercises, the special events group are probably the most important, because they should improve speed and coordination and provide variety to the program.

Lifting program

Exercise	Repetitions	Sets
Warm-up		
1. Jogging	half-mile	1
2. Flexibility exercises (98 thru 104)		
3. Sprints		
Power Exercises		
1. Modified clean (2)	10	1
2. Power press (4)	10	1
3. Squat jump (1)	10	1
Basic Exercises		
1. Dead lift (29)	15–maximum	2
2. Sit-up (26)	25–maximum to 100	2
3. Bench press (22)	10–maximum	2
4. Squat (28)	15–maximum	2
5. Overhead press (11)	10–maximum	2
6. Two-arm curl (16)	10–maximum	2
7. Tricep (17)	10–maximum	2
8. Wrist curl (20)	10–maximum	2

Lifting program (cont.)

Exercise	*Repetitions*	*Sets*

Power Rack Program (Hold each exercise approximately seven seconds)

1. Curl (33)
2. Overhead press (34)
3. Upright rowing (35)
4. Dead lift (36)
5. Bench press (37)
6. Heel-raise (38)

Supplementary Exercises

1. Rope: climbing, skipping
2. Special events: high jump, low hurdles, running and standing broad jump, sprint, vertical jump
3. Weights: incline press, lateral raise (supine), shoulder dip, shoulder press, wrist pronator, wrist roller, wall pulley exercises

DISCUSSION OF POLE VAULTING

The pole vault is probably the most difficult of all track and field events. A high premium is placed on speed, strength, agility, and coordination; so much so that the outstanding pole vaulters could probably be successful in any sport.

Right-handed jumpers carry the pole on the right side almost parallel to the ground and take off on their left foot. The position of the hand depends on the height, reach, speed, and strength of the vaulter. A good vaulter should be able to clear at least a foot higher than his grip height. During the run the pole is held loosely with the right hand close to the right hip, while the left is carried across the body, gripping the pole so that it is parallel to the ground and pointing straight down the runway.

The run must be relaxed, hitting the check marks exactly on step, and building up momentum for the vault. The run should be long enough to allow the vaulter to reach 90 to 95 percent of his maximum speed. The length of the run varies from 90 to 120 feet. Two or three strides before the takeoff the left hand begins to shift toward the right and the tip of the pole is pointed downward toward the box. The right hand should not be shifted. As the pole is planted, the hands should be no more than 3 or 4 inches apart.

The arms should be flexed at approximately 90 degrees when the pole hits the box in order to cushion the shock. The last stride before the takeoff should be slightly shorter than the previous strides so that the vaulter may gather himself for the takeoff.

The takeoff foot (left) should stamp hard on the ground as a spring up is made. The right leg is swung forward and upward as the pole is raised overhead and the arms are extended and stretched. The stomach leads the legs as the swing up is begun. As the body swings forward, the head is thrown back, the hips are swung forward and up, and the flexed right knee is turned quickly in toward the pole.

The arm pull begins only after the hips have swung up even with the shoulders and the pole is nearly vertical. The pull is made with the body close to the pole and is a quick, explosive action. It is accompanied by a body turn as the right leg drives upward.

The push-up is a continuation of the pull. The body has turned so that the stomach faces the cross bar, the arms are almost fully flexed, and the bar is against the right shoulder. While the momentum is still upward, the push-up is made so that the hips are driven upward, not away from the bar.

As the hips rise above the bar, the body is flexed at the waist and the vaulter pushes from the pole, vigorously throwing his arms over his head and away from the bar. Landing is done in a relaxed manner with the body facing the bar and the hips and knees only slightly flexed.

The muscles responsible for the take-off are primarily the leg extensors. As the pole is planted for the take-off the left leg is planted hard, causing the extensor muscles of the leg to stretch. They are then contracted powerfully as in any jumping event. The muscles of the shoulders and arms are put under full stretch during the swing. The hand flexors (flexor carpi group) tightly grasp the bar during this phase of the vault. Otherwise, the momentum is mostly the result of a sprint and jump.

When the hips have swung up almost to the height of the shoulders, the arm pull is accomplished with a powerful contraction of the shoulder girdle adductors (trapezius, rhomboids), shoulder flexors (anterior deltoid, pectoralis major), elbow flexors (biceps, brachialis), and wrist flexors (flexor carpi group). The legs are thrown up with a vigorous contraction of the hip flexors. The push-up is done primarily with the elbow extensors (triceps) and the wrist extensors (extensor carpi group). The extensor muscles of the back (quadratus lumborum, sacrospinalis) and hips (gluteus maximus) are used to extend the trunk and legs upward to their maximum height before the bar is cleared.

Probably the most important muscles for vaulting are the arm and shoulder flexors and the shoulder abductors. Obviously the athlete with powerful arms and shoulders who can easily handle his body weight with his hands has an advantage in pole vaulting. Narrow hips and small legs are advantageous if they are also strong and fast enough to build up the momentum necessary for the higher vaults. Vaulting is a delicate skill that requires a great deal of practice before proper timing and technique are mastered. However, all will go for naught if the arms and shoulders aren't properly developed.

Weight-training Program

Many coaches make a mistake in attempting to develop a vaulter over a four-month season. Actually, in order to develop a top vaulter, the training program should be a year-round one, designed to develop strength, speed, and agility, as well as vaulting technique.

The weight-training program should be designed with special emphasis on arm and shoulder strength. There is a great need for running speed and jumping spring, but care must be taken to keep down the weight of the hips and legs so that they might be more easily pushed up to maximum height. Therefore, there is only one lift suggested among the basic exercises for the legs. Although there is little probability of the legs and hips becoming bulky from the squat exercise if the vaulter continues to work at his specialty, it is suggested that the program be supplemented with vertical jumps and sprinting. It is also a good idea to perform the squats in an explosive action for maximum leg power development.

Supplementary exercises are offered using various pieces of apparatus. Any one of these can be used to vary the combined program of weight training and vaulting. There is, however, a tendency to become completely engrossed in these routine-breakers and to neglect practicing the pole vault. The only way to learn to vault is to practice the specific skill time after time. Some of the supplementary exercises should be tried on days the weights are not being lifted or as a routine-breaker for certain exercises. The vaulting practice should be completed each day before the weight-training program is begun.

Lifting program

Exercise	Repetitions	Sets
Warm-up		
1. Jogging	half-mile	1
2. Flexibility exercises (98 thru 104)		
3. Sprints	5	1
Power Exercises		
1. Modified clean (2)	10	1
2. Power press (4)	10	1
3. Squat jump (1)	10	1
4. Power curl (3)	10	1
Basic Exercises		
1. Squat (28)	15–maximum	2
2. Sit-up (26)	25–maximum to 100	2
3. Bench press (22)	10–maximum	2
4. Dead lift, Straight legs (25)	10–10	2

Lifting program (cont.)

Exercise	Repetitions	Sets
5. Straight-arm pullover (23)	10-maximum	2
6. Overhead press (11)	10-maximum	2
7. Two-arm curl (16)	10-maximum	2
8. Tricep (17)	10-maximum	2
9. Rowing (12)	10-maximum	2

Power Rack Program (Hold each exercise approximately seven seconds)
1. Curl (33)
2. Overhead press (34)
3. Upright rowing (35)
4. Bench press (37)

Supplementary Exercises
1. Flying rings: chin-up, back uprise, kip, front uprise
2. Horizontal bars: chin-up, chin-up to front support, kip
3. Mats: push-up, handstand, walk on hands, handstand push-up
4. Parallel bar: dip, front uprise, back uprise, hand balance, handstand push-up
5. Rope: climb, swing, vault
6. Weights: dead lift, forward bend, heel-raise, incline press, leg-raise, reverse curl, wrist curl

SELECTED REFERENCES

Bresnahan, George T., and W. W. Tuttle, *Track and Field Athletics,* 7th ed. St. Louis: The C. V. Mosby Company, 1969.

Doherty, J. Kenneth, *Modern Track and Field.* Englewood Cliffs, N.J.: Prentice-Hall, Inc., 1953.

Track and Field Omnibook. Swarthmore, Penna.: Tafmop Publishers, 1971.

Hoffman, Bob, *Better Athletes Through Weight Training.* York, Pa.: Strength and Health Publishing Company, 1959.

Mortensen, Jesse P., and John M. Cooper, *Track and Field for Coach and Athlete.* Englewood Cliffs, N.J.: Prentice-Hall, Inc., 1960.

Stampfl, Franz, *Franz Stampfl on Running.* New York: The Macmillan Company, 1960.

11

WEIGHT TRAINING
IN OTHER SPORTS

Although there is no athletic event in which strength cannot be used to advantage, there are many sports in which weight training is seldom used. For example, it is generally recognized that strength is one of the most important assets for success in such sports as golf and tennis. However, weight training is seldom considered for these sports. Most players have the impression that they will become strong enough by continually playing and practicing these games, not realizing that swinging an object as light as a golf club or a tennis racket doesn't bring about a great increase in strength. Unless a player has developed strength from his other activities, the chances are good that he will never be strong enough to reach his full potential in either sport.

GENERAL WEIGHT-TRAINING PROGRAM FOR ATHLETES

In this chapter a general weight-training program is presented that can be used as a point of departure for any sport. This core program can be used in its entirety with no changes, or it can be supplemented with special exercises relative to a particular sport. The program is divided into four parts: (1) warm-up, (2) power exercises, (3) basic exercises and (4) power rack isometric exercises. Special exercises for sports such as tennis or golf can be performed in a group after the warm-up and before the power exercises, or they can be interwoven into the basic program of exercises. These usually involve the small-muscle groups, such as the flexors and extensors of the wrist.

However, if additional exercises are needed for the more powerful leg and trunk muscles, they should be performed at the end of the workout, because they are very strenuous and the body requires more time for recuperation.

As has been recommended throughout this book, practice of the athletic event should precede the weight-training program if both are to be attempted on the same day. If weight training is practiced first, the muscles are too tired to accurately perform fine skills immediately afterward. Thus, it is a better idea to weight train after practice, thereby supplementing the practice session, not substituting for it.

The power rack isometric exercises offer a great opportunity to isolate specific muscle groups for strength development, and each muscle group can be exercised at different critical angles. After working with the program a few weeks, one should design exercises that will closely apply to the skill being developed to supplement the basic program.

General weight-training program for athletes

Exercise	Repetitions	Sets
Warm-up & Stretching		
1. Jogging	1 lap	1
2. Squat thrust	10	1
3. Trunk rotation	5 right, 5 left	1
4. Neck rotation	5 right, 5 left	1
5. Arm circling	5 forward, 5 backward	1
Power Exercises		
1. Modified clean (2)	10	1
2. Power curl (3)	10	1
3. Power press (4)	10	1
4. Squat jump (1)	10	1
Basic Exercises		
1. Squat (28)	15-maximum	2
2. Bench press (22)	10-maximum	2
3. Heel-raise (30)	15-maximum	2
4. Sit-up (26)	25-maximum to 100	2
5. Dead lift, Straight legs (25)	10-10	2
6. Two-arm curl (16)	10-maximum	2
7. Overhead press (11)	10-maximum	2
8. Rowing upright (13)	10-maximum	2

Power Rack Program (Hold each exercise approximately seven seconds)
1. Curl (33)
2. Overhead press (34)
3. Upright rowing (35)

General weight-training program for athletes (cont.)

Exercise	*Repetitions*	*Sets*

4. Dead lift (36)
5. Bench press (37)
6. Heel-raise (38)

In recent years some of the world's best athletes have engaged in weight training and have given credit to weights for improved performances. In a sport such as handball where one would hardly think strength to be especially important, it is noted that the 1960 National AAU champion, Jimmy Jacobs, trained with dumbbells three days a week. Other athletes have used weights to train for boxing, canoeing, cycling, rowing, soccer, water polo, and wrestling. In almost any sport that can be mentioned, some of the top performers have practiced weight training. In each of these sports the general weight-training program for athletes can be used with good results, modifying and supplementing the program with special exercises when needed.

Special emphasis has recently been placed on weight training in golf and tennis. Because they are two of the most popular recreational, as well as competitive, sports, they appear worthy of additional discussion.

Weight Training in Golf

The outstanding golfer on the professional tour in 1960 was a young man who played his college days at Wake Forest, Arnold Palmer. Not only is Palmer one of the best golfers of all time, he is one of the most muscular. Much of the credit for his phenomenal success must be attributed to his tremendous power. In recent years Jack Nicklaus has enjoyed the same advantage and has used his extra distance to dominate the game.

However, golf is one sport in which the smaller players have a chance to excel if they have very powerful wrists and hands. Jerry Barber is an excellent example of a small player overcoming the size handicap. At 137 pounds, he is one of the smallest to make the professional tour, but also one of the most successful. After particularly successful tours in 1959 and 1960 it was revealed that Barber has spent a great deal of time doing exercises, especially those that develop the arms and hands. Included in his daily exercise schedule are 120 push-ups and exercises with a 25-pound dumbbell.[1] His exercise program has given him the additional strength he needs to hit the ball out with the bigger players.

Gary Player is another golfer who isn't blessed with a large frame. Player, who has won all of the major tournaments, manages to stay around the top of

[1] Ray Cave, "A Barber with a Razor Edge," *Sports Illustrated,* (July 25, 1960), p. 42.

the list of professional money winners by performing seventy fingertip push-ups each day,[2] thereby offsetting his handicap in size.

For several years the top amateur golfer in the country was Frank Stranahan. An avid weight-lifter, Stranahan reportedly made arrangements to train with weights while traveling about the country playing tournaments. By training with very heavy weights during his playing tour, he defied all of the popular training practices. His string of amateur victories made believers of many of his critics.

There is a valid reason why a golfer must have strong hands and wrists. The distance a golf ball may be hit is dependent primarily on timing and hand and wrist strength. As the clubhead contacts the ball, the swing must be so timed that the full power of the body is thrown into the ball. The hands impart the final impetus, and it is through them that the full power of the arms, shoulders, and the rest of the body is transferred. Therefore, even though strong shoulders and a strong body are valuable, they mean little if the hands and wrists are weak.

There are several excellent exercises to strengthen the hands, wrists, and forearms. Some that are highly recommended are the Wrist Roller (41), Wrist Curl (20), Reverse Wrist Curl (21), Wrist Adduction, and the Wrist Abduction.

It is suggested that golfers substitute a specialty group of exercises in the place of a power rack program. These exercises require only improvised equipment and the group makes up a good alternate-day program which can be used by the amateur or the touring professional. The program listed below has incorporated this idea.

Weight-training program for golf

Exercise	Repetitions	Sets
Warm-up & Stretching		
1. Jogging	1 lap	1
2. Squat thrust	10	1
3. Trunk rotation	5 right, 5 left	1
4. Arm circling	5 forward, 5 backward	1
Power Exercises		
1. Modified clean (2)	10	1
2. Power curl (3)	10	1
3. Power press (4)	10	1
4. Squat jump (1)	10	1
Basic Exercises		
1. Squat (28)	15	1

[2]*The Winston-Salem Journal,* (March 27, 1961), p. 11.

Weight-training program for golf (cont.)

Exercise	Repetitions	Sets
2. Bench press (22)	10-maximum	2
3. Sit-up (26)	25-25	2
4. Dead lift, Straight legs (25)	10-10	2
5. Two-arm curl (16)	10-maximum	2
6. Overhead press (11)	10-maximum	2
7. Rowing upright (13)	10-maximum	2
8. Wrist curl (20)	10	1
Specialty Exercises		
1. Chinning	Maximum	1
2. Sit-up	Maximum	1
3. Push-up	Maximum	1
4. Dips	Maximum	1

Weight Training in Tennis

For a number of years the Australian tennis players were the best in the world. Although in this country little is heard of weight training for tennis, a large percentage of the Australian players have trained regularly with weights, including such stars as Frank Sedgman, Lew Hoad, Ashley Cooper, Ken McGregor, Ken Rosewall, and Neale Fraser.[3] Sedgman has operated a training gym in Melbourne.

The training program practiced by the Australians reportedly calls for a variety of exercises designed to improve strength and agility. Many of the exercises with the wall pulley and dumbbells closely imitate tennis strokes. Above all, however, the program calls for a lot of tennis practice. Such a training program gave the Australian players a terrific advantage over the players in the United States, most of whom trained by playing only. Even though the comparative skills may be near equal, the superior strength and power of the Australians prevailed until both began using similar training programs.

Many of the same exercises recommended for golf should be practiced by tennis players. In addition, the tennis player should engage in a variety of arm and shoulder exercises that resemble the action of tennis strokes. Some of the best exercises are the Tricep (17), Lateral Raise, Supine (24), Straight-Arm Pullover (23), Bent-Arm Pullover, Shoulder Dips (19), and Chinning (18).

Competitive tennis is practically a year-round sport for many players. There are many high school and college players, however, who have little

[3]Ray Van Cleef, "Winning Tennis Via Weights," *Strength and Health* (July 1958), p. 44.

opportunity to compete during the winter months. They should spend at least two or three of the winter months training with weights. During the playing season they should practice the special exercises for the hands and wrists almost daily.

The modern tennis champions play the big game, featuring aggressive play with booming serves and drives. These players are exceptional athletes; strong, agile, and well-coordinated. Finesse and skill may compensate for a lack of strength in some high school and college circles, but in better tennis tournaments the winner is usually the player with strength as well as skill.

The weight-training program for tennis shown below is a basic program which lends itself to amateur or professional. On alternate days it is very important to use the specialty exercises, or similar ones.

Weight-training program for tennis

Exercise	*Repetitions*	*Sets*
Warm-up & Stretching		
1. Jogging	1 lap	1
2. Squat thrust	10	1
3. Trunk rotation	5 right, 5 left	1
4. Arm circling	5 forward, 5 backward	1
Power Exercises		
1. Modified clean (2)	10	1
2. Power curl (3)	10	1
3. Power press (4)	10	1
4. Squat jump (1)	10	1
Basic Exercises		
1. Squat (28)	15	1
2. Bench press (22)	10-maximum	2
3. Sit-up (26)	25-maximum to 100	2
4. Dead lift, Straight legs (25)	10-10	2
5. Two-arm curl (16)	10-maximum	2
6. Overhead press (11)	10-maximum	2
7. Rowing upright (13)	10-maximum	2
8. Wrist curl (20)	10-maximum	2
9. Straight-arm pullover (23)	10-maximum	2
Specialty Exercises		
1. Chinning	maximum	1
2. Push-up	maximum	1
3. Lateral raise, supine	maximum	1
4. Dips	maximum	1

12

WEIGHT TRAINING IN PHYSICAL EDUCATION

Now that the barrier of superstition which for years has been associated with lifting weights is at last being lifted, it is rapidly gaining an important place in the school and college physical education programs across the nation as a supplement to activity courses or as a complete course covering an entire semester. In recent years the physical fitness of our youth has become so poor that drastic steps are needed to cope with the problem. Current physical education programs are partly responsible for the dilemma. Since World War II, the majority of programs have been geared to a wide range of social and recreational type activities, with little or no emphasis on physical development or fitness. It is anticipated that these programs of sports education will so interest the students in physical activity that they will retain this interest and participate in sports long after they graduate from school. Such has been the case with only a very small percentage, however; and of those who continue to exercise, most play sports of a nonvigorous nature.

The modern philosophy of sports education is good, but it is not meeting the needs of the American people. It is based on the idea that one can play his way into good physical condition. As one gets older this practice becomes more and more difficult and dangerous. Therefore, the program of sports education should be supplemented with a program of weight training or some comparative conditioning exercises that overload all of the major muscle groups of the body and subject them to vigorous exercise. A combination of the two programs should be inaugurated in schools so that our students will be better able to participate in and enjoy all sports. They should learn early that the proper procedure is to condition to play, because they will not always be able to play to condition.

A BRIEF HISTORY OF WEIGHT TRAINING

In its earliest form, lifting was an essential for daily living; but the exact period in history when the practice of lifting weights actually started is not known. There is evidence of some lifting contests to satisfy the competitive urges of man long before the Christian era. History tells of some forms of lifting contests and demonstrations by the Greeks and Egyptians in those ancient days. There is also evidence of early forms of weight training for the purpose of developing better fighting men, and it is probable that the first organized training programs existed to develop the soldiers of that day.

References to weight lifting appear frequently in European history, but until the nineteenth century little is known about its popularity and acceptance. During the early part of that century the Turnverein movement was established in Germany by Dr. Frederick Jahn. He advocated special clubs for specific physical activity, one of which included weight training with dumbbells. These clubs were highly active and successful throughout the country and did much to popularize conditioning with weights.

Weight training was brought to the United States by immigrants from many foreign countries. Although the Austrian, Swiss, and French immigrants practiced with weights, the real impetus was provided by the Germans with their Turnverein clubs scattered across the United States. By the middle of the nineteenth century, lifting weights was well established in this country.

Around the turn of the twentieth century, the primary purpose of weight lifting apparently was theatrical entertainment. Many men and women alike were performing spectacular feats of strength in carnivals, circuses, and theaters. This practice continued until recent years and has probably been responsible for much of the reluctance with which weight training is being accepted by the American people. Many of the entertainers built their spectacular acts around trickery and deceit, and even though some fantastic feats of strength were recorded during this period, many of them were obviously spectacular misrepresentations.

Weight lifting gradually found its way into the athletic clubs, and in recent years the YMCAs have continually promoted the competitive sport of weight lifting in their activity program. The Amateur Athletic Union of the United States included weight lifting as a sport in their program of competition and held the first American National Championships in 1929. In 1932 the United States entered its first team in the Olympic games, and in 1948 won the championship for the first time.

Growth of weight training in recent years has been extraordinary. There are several good reasons for this:

1. Research has continued to dispel the doubts and superstitions surrounding the activity and has proven it to be a safe method of building strength, power, and endurance.

2. Lifting programs were used with excellent results during and after World War II in Army and Navy hospitals for the rehabilitation of the injured.

3. More recently, weight training has been used successfully to strengthen the muscles, thereby helping to prevent injuries in sports.

4. Weight training has been used very successfully to help improve specific athletic abilities.

More and more schools and colleges are recognizing the values to be derived from lifting weights, and by redirecting the emphasis from competitive lifting to a systematic method of exercising with weights, they are deriving many extra benefits. Weight training, as it is usually referred to in the physical education programs, is rapidly gaining recognition, and conceivably in a few years will be an accepted part of every high school and college program.

LIFTING PROGRAMS

There are probably as many different types of weight training programs in physical education classes as there are schools offering such courses. This doesn't mean that there isn't a right way and a wrong way to train with weights. What it does mean is that training with weights has many values, and a good program may necessarily go in serveral directions to fulfill the objectives of the course. A program may be directed primarily toward conditioning and body-building with special emphasis on strength. It may be a program in which competitive lifting is stressed and the total amount of weight lifted using the three Olympic lifts is the main objective. It can be designed to correct or improve physical disabilities. Or possibly the course objectives may be aimed toward all three areas. The important thing is to outline the objectives and to design and conduct the training program with those objectives clearly in focus.

Much has been said in previous sections about facilities, equipment, and time allotment. The program must also be made to conform to the lifting area, the number of sets of weights, and the amount of time available. Therefore, it cannot be too strongly emphasized that the program be made to fit the situation, not the situation to fit the program.

Training programs suggested in this book apply to most situations. If not, they can probably be suitably altered with little difficulty. If none of the programs can be used, you may wish to design your own. In that event, the following considerations are also important:

1. Including resistive exercises for all of the major muscle groups of the body

2. Including in each program some exercises that incorporate a full body movement

3. Arranging the exercises so that muscle groups are allowed to rest between lifting sets
4. Maintaining variety in the program
5. Being enthusiastic — if it's worth doing at all, it's worth doing well

Basic Weight-training Unit

The primary purpose for the actual lifting phase of the weight-training unit should be to improve general physical strength and fitness. To accomplish this it is necessary to exercise all of the muscle groups, with a particular emphasis on the muscles of the arms and shoulders. A very good program is one similar to that made popular by Bob Hoffman,[1] which calls for a medium program on Monday, a light program on Wednesday, and a heavy program on Friday. We have experienced much success with a similar program using a "regular 10-maximum program" on Monday, a "variety program" on Wednesday, in which a large number of exercises are performed only one set each with a relatively light weight, and a "heavy program" on Friday using a low number of repetitions with heavy weights. Such a program ensures maximum strength gains and general physical fitness. To further improve fitness we require a number of running excercises. This program is incorporated into the following unit of instruction.

This program differs slightly from the program described in other sections of this book because of the lifting time available in each session. It is assumed that in a physical education class there will be only thirty to thirty-five minutes of actual lifting time. Therefore, the programs for Wednesday and Friday differ. The variety program on Wednesday is a great routine-breaker and teaches additional lifts to the class members. The heavy program on Friday is a "6-maximum-maximum" program, adding weight with each set after starting the first set with six repetitions. The first set for each lift should usually be performed with the same weight used on the last set on Monday.

Teaching Unit

Physical education units may involve any number of class sessions. The following unit covers an entire semester of 45 class sessions meeting 50 minutes every other day. It is offered as a guide or a point of departure for physical education teachers who plan to teach a basic course of weight training. We have been very pleased with the enthusiastic acceptance of a similar program.

[1]*Better Athletes Through Weight Training,* York, Pa.: Strength and Health Publishing Co., (1959); p. 92.

Unit Objectives:

1. Improving general body strength and appearance
2. Developing physical fitness through a general conditioning program
3. Teaching the theoretical aspects: the "why," "how," and "benefits" of weight training
4. Developing skill in the proper execution of the various lifts and a knowledge of what muscles are involved
5. Encouraging improvement through self-competition and through competition with other class members
6. Making the training program enjoyable by providing variety and recognizing and praising progress
7. Developing an appreciation of weight training as an enjoyable way to keep physically fit

Reading:

Before attempting to teach a weight-training unit of instruction read chapters 2, 3, 4 and 5 carefully. If the unit is planned for a specific situation, these chapters should be referred to as frequently as necessary.

Session one, Monday

I. Why condition?
   A. Present generation
      1. Mechanization of our society is almost complete
      2. Result is an overfed and underworked musculature
   B. Breakdown areas of the body
      1. Abdominal area expands and weakens
         (a) Posture deteriorates
         (b) Circulation impaired
      2. Foot trouble is caused by excess weight, poor muscle tone, and poor walking habits
      3. Strength declines
         (a) Body loses ability to handle ordinary emergencies
         (b) There is no reserve energy to enjoy living after work
   C. General need for adequate strength
      1. Responsibility to self to avoid physical degeneration
      2. Responsibility to family
      3. Responsibility to country
II. Benefits of weight training
   A. Strength
      1. Muscle fibers strengthen and enlarge

  2. Quality of muscular contraction improves

  3. Muscle functions with more power and less effort

 B. Endurance

  1. Improves ability to make a sustained effort

 C. Posture

  1. Physique is built by weight training

  2. Good posture and carriage usually accompany strength

 D. Circulation

  1. Conditioned heart does more work with fewer beats

  2. Venous and capillary circulation can be improved

 E. Vital organs and glands

  1. Body thrives on function

  2. Digestion, assimilation, absorption, and elimination improve

 F. Mental health

  1. Encourages release of tension and induces fatigue and relaxation

Session two, Wednesday

I. How to condition

 A. Physiological facts indicate fitness necessary for complete living

  1. Overload principle

   (a) Strength and enlargement of muscle results from use if resistance is gradually increased to the maximum

   (b) Endurance is improved best by increasing the number of movements; muscular endurance is associated with an increase in capillaries and strength, cardiorespiratory endurance is primarily a development of "wind."

  2. "Underload principle"

   (a) Disuse of muscles results in weakness, malfunction, and atrophy (wasting away)

  3. Muscular size and strength

   (a) Strength of muscle is proportional to its effective cross-section

   (b) Short bouts of vigorous exercise build muscle faster

  4. Maintenance

   (a) Strength can be maintained with one or two workouts a week

   (b) Endurance requires a daily effort

  5. Psychological limits

   (a) Limits are pain, fear, aches, and respiratory discomfort

   (b) Psychological limits are reached long before physiological limits

   (c) Competition and desire for social approval help raise psychological limit

B. Individual needs

    1. Ability to recuperate after exercise is an excellent guide to proper conditioning

    2. Condition gradually before maximum efforts

       (a) To insure against injury and physical torment go slowly for two to three weeks

Session three, Friday

I. Class organization

  A. Class size and time available

    1. This plan can be adjusted to accommodate as many boys as there are weights available. Ideally the class size is twenty-four, four to each set of weights. Larger numbers may be accommodated by increasing the number of boys to each set of weights to five, or by getting additional sets and adding more lifting stations.

       If the multiple-use machine is used, the number will depend entirely on the number of stations the machine has. Some have as many as ten or eleven. It is very difficult to use more than six at one time, four boys to each station.

    2. This plan is designed for a fifty-minute class, thirty-five minutes of actual lifting time. For those classes that meet every day, the Tuesday and Thursday sessions can best be devoted to cross-country, relay races, or other running games.

  B. Equipment

    1. A barbell plus 75 pounds of plates are needed for high school boys at each lifting station. College freshmen need at least 100 pounds of plates. An area 7 feet square is needed for each lifting station. A multiple-use machine may be used. It should have at least six stations. If two are used, twice as many students may be accommodated, but the organization and administration of the class is quite difficult.

    2. If the gym floor is used, a mat such as a large rubber door mat should be placed at each station to protect the floor. Arrange the stations as the facilities permit, using the diagram in Figure 9 as a guide.

    3. A bench should be located at each station if possible

    4. Dumbbells can be used if available

  C. Grading

    1. Discuss with class how their grades will be determined

       (a) Strength and fitness

       (b) Skill

        (c) Improvement

        (d) Knowledge

        (e) Social efficiency

    D. Nomenclature

        1. Explanation and demonstration of lifting grips

           (a) Overhand

           (b) Underhand

           (c) Alternate

        2. Explanation and demonstration of lifting positions (using weight sets or multiple-use machine, whichever is appropriate)

           (a) Standing

           (b) Crouch

           (c) Thigh rest

           (d) Chest rest

           (e) Shoulder rest

           (f) Prone

           (g) Supine

        3. Explanation and demonstration of counting weight

        4. Health and safety practices

           (a) Medical examination

           (b) Lifting precautions

           (c) Use of warm-up

           (d) Avoidance of chilling

           (e) Avoidance of horseplay

           (f) Avoidance of hernia

           (g) Proper diet

           (h) Sleep

    E. Class procedure

        1. Explanation of procedure in setting weights out and putting them away

        2. Grouping

           (a) Maximum lifts to determine relative strength

           (b) According to size

         3. Practice with light weight the lifting grips and positions

           (a) Rotation

           (b) Spotting

           (c) Changing weight

Session four, Monday

I. Lifting program

    A. Warm-up exercises

     1. Jogging

     2. Squat thrust

     3. Trunk and neck rotation

     4. Arm circling

B. Demonstration of each lift accompanied by brief lecture on muscles exercised.

C. Performance of each lift. The trainers should perform each lift one set of ten repetitions with very light weight; probably from 35 to 50 pounds. The instructor should circulate from station to station to criticize

     1. Power exercises (only for those using conventional sets of weights)

       (a) Modified clean (2)

       (b) Power curl (3)

       (c) Squat jump (1)

       (d) Power press (4)

     2. Basic exercises (exercises b and g are not designed for the multiple-use machine. Substitute a toe-touch exercise for the Dead lift, Straight legs, and a deltoid exercise for the Rowing upright.)

       (a) Squat (28)

       (b) Dead lift, Straight legs (25)

       (c) Bench press (22)

       (d) Sit-up (26)

       (e) Overhead press (11)

       (f) Two-arm curl (16)

       (g) Rowing upright (13)

Session five, Wednesday

I. Lifting program same as Session Four

A. Perform two sets of each exercise

B. Lecture on progression

     1. Record forms should be provided for each boy and a pencil placed at each station

     2. Fill out the weight loads for each exercise to be lifted on Friday

     3. Explain that on Friday two sets of each basic exercise will be performed ten repetitions, increasing the weight 10 pounds with the second set

Session six, Friday

I. Lifting program same as Session Four

A. Perform one set of the power exercises

B. Perform the 10-10 routine of basic exercises

C. Check to see if the progression plan is understood

Session seven, Monday

I. Lifting program same as Session Four

A. Perform one set of the power exercises

B. Perform the 10-10 routine of basic exercises

C. No progression

Session eight, Wednesday

I. Same as Session Seven

Session nine, Friday

I. Same as Session Eight

A. Progress with basic exercises by adding 10 pounds to each set of an exercise when second set can be performed ten repetitions

B. Gradually increase the weight for the power exercises

C. Substitute Dead lift exercise (29) for Dead lift, Straight legs (25)

Session ten, Monday

I. Same as Session Nine, except perform the second set of each exercise the maximum number. If the maximum number exceeds 10, increase the weight for the first set for the next regular lifting session.

Session eleven, Wednesday

I. Same as Session Nine

Session twelve, Friday

I. Same as Session Nine

Session thirteen, Monday

I. Same as Session Nine

Session fourteen, Wednesday

I. Variety day

A. Same warm-up

B. Load 40 to 50 pounds on the bar and lift with explosive action

C. Perform only one set of ten repetitions of the following exercises in the order listed:

1. Modified clean (2)

2. Power curl (3)

3. Squat (28)
4. Power press (4)
5. High pull-up (6)
6. Squat (28)
7. Rowing (12)
8. Two-arm curl (16)
9. Overhead press (11)
10. Dead lift, Straight legs (25)
11. Triceps (17)
12. Knee-bend and shoulder press (7)
13. Sit-up (26)
14. Neck flexion and extension (8, 9)
15. Bench press (22)
16. Squat (28)

Session fifteen, Friday

I. Heavy day
  A. Same warm-up and power exercises
  B. Perform a 6-maximum-maximum routine of basic exercises. Start the first set of each exercise with the weight of the usual second set. Add 10 pounds for each additional set as for the 10-maximum-maximum program.

Session sixteen, Monday

I. Same as Session Thirteen

Session seventeen, Wednesday

I. Same as Session Fourteen

Session eighteen, Friday

I. Maximum lift day
  A. Same warm-up
  B. Start with the weight of the usual third set and perform only one repetition. Add weight and continue to perform one repetition until the maximum lift for each exercise has been determined. It should be reached within three or four lifts.

Session nineteen, Monday

I. Same as Session Thirteen

Session twenty, Wednesday

I. Same as Session Fourteen

Session twenty-one, Friday

I. Same as Session Fifteen

Session twenty-two, Monday

I. Divide the class into interest groups
  A. Those who wish should be allowed to substitute the three competitive lifts for the established routine on Wednesdays and Fridays
  B. The others may continue the same routine of Regular Day, Variety Day, and Heavy Day

Session twenty-three, Wednesday

I. Regular group
  A. Continue established routine
II. Competitive group
  A. Discuss general rules
  B. Demonstrate and discuss the execution of the lifts
    1. Two-hand military press
    2. Two-hand snatch
    3. Two-hand clean and jerk
  C. Practice with light weight

Session twenty-four, Friday

I. Regular group
  A. Continue established routine
II. Competitive group
  A. Practice the competitive lifts

Session twenty-five, Monday

I. Regular group
  A. Continue established routine
II. Competitive group
  A. Work with regular group

Session twenty-six, Wednesday

I. Regular group
  A. Continue established routine
II. Competitive group
  A. Practice the competitive lifts, gradually increasing the weight loads

Session twenty-seven through session forty-three

I. Continue designated routines

Session forty-four, Wednesday

I. Written exam on weight training

Session forty-five, Friday

I. Maximum lift day
II. Turn in all record Sheets

Competitive Lifting

There is great value to be derived from competitive lifting. However, it should not be substituted for a basic weight-training unit or for another activity unit of a physical education class unless the boys are first adequately conditioned and trained in lifting. Only then should they be allowed to concentrate on the three Olympic lifts. An ideal way to include competitive lifting in the program is to make it a part of the complete course as illustrated in the unit of instruction.

The Olympic barbell used for competitive lifting differs considerably from the standard weight training equipment. The bar is 7 feet long and has a revolving sleeve at each end where the weights attach. The bar and collars weigh 55 pounds, 30 pounds more than the standard sets. The plates are also different sizes, and shapes, graduated upward, in the following poundages: 2½, 5, 10, 25, 35, and 45. Lifts in actual contests are done on a wooden platform approximately 12 feet square.

There are three recognized lifts: the two-hand military press, the two-hand snatch, and the two-hand clean and jerk. Each competitor is allowed three trials for each lift, or a total of nine lifts in a contest. Between each trial the increase of weight must not be less than 10 pounds except the last one, which may be 5 pounds. An increase of 5 pounds on any trial denotes the last try for that lift. The lifter may not carry out a trial with a lighter weight than that employed in the previous trial. Each competitor must determine for himself the weight with which he wishes to begin. When he fails to complete a lift, the judges shall allow him a maximum rest of three minutes before the next trial. If he is unsuccessful with his first or second attempts, he may try again with the same weight. In case of a tie, the lighter man wins.

There are three officials, a referee and two judges, to determine the correctness of each trial. In case of disagreement the majority rules. The referee also must decide when the lifter has the bar under control and must signal when it may be lowered. The signal to start a press is a clap of the hands. To lower the bar, the signal is a downward wave and a shout of "down." Signals must be obvious.

The totals made by the lifters on their best successful efforts on the three lifts determine the winners in the seven bodyweight classes. These classes are as follows:

Bantamweight	123 1/4	Lightheavyweight		181 3/4
Featherweight	132 1/4	Middleheavyweight		198 1/4
Lightweight	148 3/4	Heavyweight	over	198 1/4
Middleweight	165 1/4			

The rules for and the techniques of the three Olympic lifts are described generally in the following pages. For those who are interested in competitive lifting as an extracurricular activity, more detailed information concerning the rules may be obtained by writing the Amateur Athletic Union (AAU). For information regarding proper technique the outstanding authority in America is the former coach of the American Olympic weight lifting team, Bob Hoffman. His book *Guide to Weight Lifting Competition* is an excellent training guide.

Because only a little time is available in physical education classes to train for Olympic lifting, the following teaching points are suggested:

1. Teach the clean and press, clean and jerk, and snatch, in the order listed.
2. Start by teaching form with relatively light weight.
3. Do not attempt to break down the lifts into parts for teaching purposes. Teach the fully coordinated movement of each lift and require the students to exhibit reasonably good form in each lift before allowing them to increase the weight.
4. As specific weaknesses persist, correct them by improving techniques or by recommending special exercises to build the inhibiting muscle groups.
5. Remember there are four primary reasons why boys choose to work with weights: (1) pleasures of weight lifting itself, (2) body-building, (3) weight training for athletics, and (4) rehabilitation. It is a teacher's duty to attempt to provide the opportunity for a boy to reach his maximum potential in either of the four. If a boy develops interest in competitive lifting, an outlet should be provided for it if possible. Such interest can best be cultivated through weight-lifting clubs and interscholastic teams.

Two-hand Military Press

Grasp the bar with an overhand grip and clean it to the chest rest position. The feet should be on the same line and no more than 16 inches apar

Mark a two-second stop, standing motionless in this position. Slowly press the bar up until the arms are completely extended overhead. There should be no jerk or sudden start in the press. Hold the overhead position for two seconds, both arms and legs extended. During the entire execution of the press the body must be kept vertical.

In competition the bar must usually touch the chest before the second movement is started, and the bar is not lowered until the referee signals. If the lifter can't touch the bar to his chest he should inform the judges before the lift. The lifter is disqualified if the head and body do not maintain the vertical position, if there is any twisting or bending of the body, if there is any foot motion or bending of the legs, if the arms are extended unevenly, or if the barbell is lowered slightly before the press.

There are various special techniques to pressing that some lifters have found advantageous. The two most important ones are: (1) maintaining a good foundation position with the hips thrust forward, the legs locked and the chest raised high; and (2) pressing up and back from the chest, keeping the bar close to the face.

Some of the best lifters employ what is called the thumbless grip in pressing. This means that the thumbs are placed behind the bar with the fingers

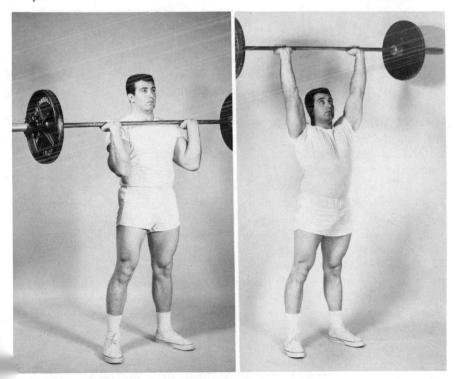

Figure 73. Two-hand Military Press

instead of gripping around it. Those who use this grip contend that it enables them to concentrate all of their strength in the upward drive of the bar and that none of it is wasted in gripping. The hands are usually placed slightly wider than shoulder-width.

Two-hand Snatch

The simplest lift to describe, but the most difficult to perform, is the two-hand snatch. The barbell must be lifted from a crouch position in a single, continuous motion to fully locked arms overhead. The lifter is allowed to duck under the bar as long as the upward motion of the bar isn't interrupted and provided neither knee touches the floor. The lift is disqualified if there is a break in the upward motion, if the lifter can't stay on the platform, or if the bar can't be held overhead for the entire two-second count.

The most basic fundamental in the snatch is the one-motion pull from the floor to the arms overhead position. The lifter should stand so close to the bar that his shins almost touch, with the head up, the back flat, and the hips low. Using an overhand grip, usually with the thumbs hooked under the fingers and the hands wider than shoulder-width, he should pull the bar as close to the body as possible. The pull must be started with the legs and as momentum is gained the arms and back must pull powerfully. The next impetus is given with the legs by a rise on the toes, while at the same time the wrists and hands flip under the bar. Finally, the body dips under, the arms are locked overhead, and the lifter stands erect with the arms and legs fully extended.

There are two techniques for performing the snatch, the squat and the split. In the squat the lifter is able to duck his weight under the bar by splitting his legs apart and sitting to a full knee bend postion, simultaneously catching the weight overhead. The head should be thrust forward with the shoulders retracted. He completes the lift by standing erect with the weight under control and with the feet on the same line. The squat may be the best method to snatch so far as power is concerned, but maintaining balance is much more difficult than in the split style.

With the split technique, the snatch is performed in the same way as in the squat, except that as the lifter ducks under the bar one leg extends behind with the knee slightly flexed, the weight falling on the ball of the foot. The other leg thrusts forward with the knee considerably bent and the foot flat on the floor.

Two-hand clean and jerk

This lift is performed in two separate movements: (1) the bar is cleaned to the chest-rest position; and (2) the bar is jerked to the arms overhead position. The bar must be held under control overhead for two seconds, or until the referee signals. The clean to the shoulders is performed as described for the two-hand military press. It must be a continuous movement from the platform to the chest-rest postition. When the bar has been properly positioned at the chest-rest position the feet must be brought to a straight line with the legs extended. The second movement of the lift is to power the bar to an arm locked overhead position. This is done by bending the knees and hips ar

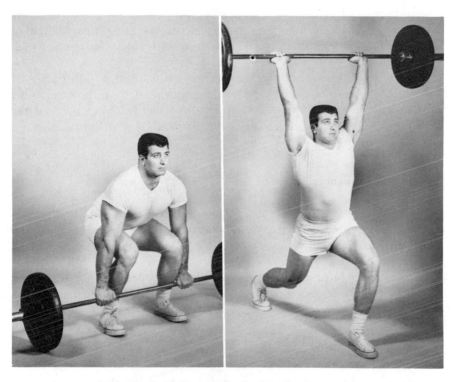

Figure 74. Two-hand Snatch, Split Style

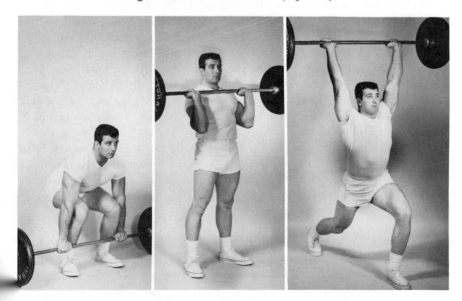

Figure 75. Two-hand Clean and Jerk, Split Style

powerfully extending them, at the same time powering the bar overhead by extending the arms. The lifter then ducks under the bar using either the split or squat. The final movement involves coming to an erect position by stepping back with the front leg.

It is against the rules if the knee touches the platform in either phase; if the bar touches any part of the body while bringing it from the floor to the chest rest position; if the elbows touch the knees during the clean; or if the overhead position is not held for a two-second count. A second attempt is not permitted if the first jerk is successful.

Special Programs

Weight-training units in high school and college physical education programs may proceed in a number of directions, depending primarily on the leadership, facilities, and equipment available. Although the usual procedure is to offer a basic course in general conditioning and strengthening, it is a popular practice in some high schools to use the physical education class period for training an athletic squad. Weights are also being used more and more in the rehabilitation of injuries.

Athletics

Certainly there can be no better activity for an athlete than lifting weights. All evidence on the subject has proven this to be true beyond any doubt. Although there is no objection to an athlete training with weights during physical education classes to improve his athletic ability, it should be done after school hours if it restricts the weight-training facilities from use by the rest of the student body. Physical education classes are for all students, and all courses should be offered to them so far as facilities, equipment, and scheduling will permit. Weight training in physical education classes, by the same token, should be for all students, especially those who do not get the benefit of participating in the varsity athletic program.

Occasionally it might be possible that an entire athletic squad be scheduled in a physical education class. If this can be done with no special inconvenience to the rest of the classes, the weight-training programs described for the different sports can be used. They can be shortened when there is such a need by reducing the number of sets for each exercise.

The most frequent method of offering weight training to athletes during physical education programs probably comes as an outgrowth of the basic conditioning program. The program is arranged so that after the players have participated in a basic conditioning program with the other class members, they are permitted to participate in a weight program specifically designed to improve their specialties. The programs for various sports must be worked out by the instructor, using the apppropriate chapters in this book as a guide.

As a rule, it isn't a very good idea for an instructor to spread himself too thin. It is practically impossible to conduct lifting programs for athletes, competitive lifting programs, basic programs, and rehabilitation programs all at once. However, if the class is small enough and facilities and equipment are adequate, the basic program and the athletic program can be conducted together successfully.

Physical Disabilities

The most neglected students in physical education classes are usually the physically handicapped. Their activity is often limited to scorekeeping and managing equipment. The terrific burden of duties and responsibilities placed on a large percentage of teachers and coaches makes it impossible to offer them more. However, in some way schools should make provisions for these students. Weight training is the logical answer for many schools who are doing nothing to provide these students with wholesome exercise. Our most satisfying weight-training programs have been for these students. Training with weights is one way that they can enjoy the thrill of physical competition; and many of them can improve their physical performance, often dramatically. They should not be deprived of such an opportunity.

No physical education instructor has the right to design and supervise weight training for a handicapped student until the program has been approved by a trained physician. The student should have a complete medical examination before anything else is done. After such an examination the program should be worked out in accordance with the recommendations of the physician, the enthusiasm and capabilities of the student, and the facilities and equipment available to the instructor at a time when he can free himself to supervise the program.

At the first class meeting the student should be asked to write a research paper on the nature of his injury, how it was incurred, the treatment, the rehabilitation program, if any, and its current status. Such a paper serves a double purpose. First, it requires the student to better understand the physical limitations of his disability. Second, it gives the instructor a better knowledge of the injury and helps him gain a deeper insight into the attitude of the student concerning the injury.

There might be a strong objection by the high school student to prepare a research paper on such a personal subject. In such cases it is best to work out a weight training program without this information. However, extreme caution is recommended in designing such a program. The college age student, on the other hand, will usually be more willing to discuss and research his disability and to participate in a program which might lead to its improvement.

Many disabled students can be helped through weight training and other resistive exercises. Some of our disabled group have been victims of poliomyelitis. An increasing number have been involved in automobile accidents. Others have received their injuries while participating in athletics. The polio patients can often develop their arms and shoulders or legs through weight training to the extent that they can maneuver and handle their body weight with much more authority and confidence. Students with broken bones or sprained joints can speed the process of recovery and usually make the recovery much more complete. Atrophy of muscles can be held to a minimum.

No two disabilities are exactly alike. Even if they are almost identical, the physical make-up of individuals and their attitude toward recovery are different, affecting the design of their program. Each individual must be consulted separately and his program designed according to his individual needs.

Complete coverage of corrective exercises is not possible in this book. However, we are fortunate that there are a number of good books available on corrective exercises and adaptive programs which describe step by step procedures to follow in the rehabilitation of all types of disabilities. No matter how closely book procedures apply to a certain disability, a physician must be consulted before the responsibility for the exercise program is assumed.

GRADING

Grades for a unit in weight training should be arrived at in much the same manner as in other activity classes, and should conform with the marking system of the school administration. It is usual procedure to determine weight-training grades in relation to the objectives that have been formulated for the course. These objectives are usually grouped under three main areas, physical, mental, and social. Because the primary emphasis is on the physical element, it carries 60 percent of the grade. The mental element carries 20 percent, and the social element is valued at 20 percent.

Physical Grade — 60 Percent

The physical grade is the most important and most difficult to determine fairly. It is a common mistake to award this grade only on the basis of strength. If this is done, the weaker students will be driven off because they will not have a chance to earn a satisfactory grade. These students need weight training the most, and the grading procedure should not unduly discourage them. The physical grade should consider strength, but other factors, such as physical fitness, skill in performing lifts, and improvement in strength and appearance are also important and deserve consideration. A satisfactory plan is to weight the items for the physical grade as follows:

Strength and fitness   50%
Skill in performing lifts   25%
Improvement in strength   25%

There are very few printed norms for determining a satisfactory strength grade based solely on weight-training performance. Certainly standards are not available for all age groups and body weights. Until such standards are formulated, the most practical procedure is to combine the physical fitness and strength elements. Both are considered in most tests of fitness. The most suitable we have used is a four-item test of muscular strength and endurance. It can be easily and quickly administered indoors and in one class period. The tests should be given in the order listed so that everyone has an equal opportunity to score well.

Wake Forest fitness test

A. Pull-ups
1. To test arm flexors and shoulder strength.
2. The student must grip the bar with an underhand grip. Arms must be fully extended and the feet held above the floor. The student must pull himself up until his chin is above the horizontal bar and then let himself down until both arms are fully extended. This exercise is to be repeated for the maximum number of executions.

B. Shoulder dips
1. To test arm extensors and shoulder strength.
2. The student must grip the parallel bars and extend both arms until the elbow joints are locked. The test is executed by having the student lower his body until the elbows are bent 90 degrees and then return to the starting position. This exercise is to be repeated for a maximum number of executions.

C. Bent-knee sit-ups
1. To test trunk strength and endurance.
2. The student must lie flat on the floor with his legs spread in a comfortable position. The heels of both feet will be placed near the buttocks with the soles of both feet flat on the floor. The hands are clasped behind his head. The student will be assisted by having someone hold his feet flat on the floor. To begin this exercise the student will raise his trunk until he can touch his right elbow to his left knee and then lower his trunk to the starting position. On the second count the student will touch his left elbow to his right knee. This exercise will be repeated for a maximum number of executions within two minutes.

D. Squat jump
1. To test leg strength, power and endurance.

2. The student must begin this exercise in a full squat with one leg placed in a forward position. The fingers of both hands will be clasped on top of the student's head. He will begin by jumping into the air and extending both legs. Before returning to the squatting position the student will reverse his legs by placing the forward leg to the rear and the other leg forward. This exercise is to be repeated for the maximum number of executions.

The test has been administered to all boys in the freshman class and to all students participating in the elective course in weight training for two years. On the basis of their scores, the following norms have been set:

Fitness and strength test norms

	Pull-ups	Shoulder Dips	Bent-Knee Sit-ups	Squat Jumps
A	16 up	18 up	88 up	92 up
B	12-15	13-17	66-87	70-91
C	7-11	7-12	49-65	48-69
D	3-6	2-6	33-48	26-47
F	2 and below	1 and below	32 and below	25 and below

These norms will not apply to all age groups. However, they can be used satisfactorily as a guide for grading until T-scores can be worked out and norms established to fit your local situation.

Lifting skill and improvement can be more easily determined. Lifting skill is necessarily a subjective grade. The descriptions of the lifts in Chapter 5 should be consulted frequently for instructional and grading purposes.

Improvement in strength can be easily determined by administering a fitness and strength test during the first few days of class and readministering the test at the end of the unit. Another method is to have the students perform maximum lifts during the first few class periods and again at the end of the unit. With either way, improvement in strength can be readily determined.

Knowledge — 20 Percent

Weight training is not easy. A strong body requires a great deal of hard work and very few people will continue if they don't know what the effects will be. Therefore, it is especially important that all students be taught the theory behind weight training. They should be made aware of the values derived by a conscientious student from a good program. They should also know exactly how each lift should be performed and the specific muscle groups that are involved. Theoretical aspects of weight training should be taught during class periods wi periodic lectures and daily criticisms. A mid-term test and a final examination should be administered to determine this part of the grade.

Social — 20 Percent

The third area of grading is in social efficiency. In this area are included such traits as attitude, enthusiasm, effort, appearance, and care of equipment and facilities. Such traits are impossible to measure objectively, and consequently it is very difficult to assign a grade. A number of score cards are available for social evaluation, but at best the evaluation is a subjective rating of each trait by the instructor.

Grading Chart

Just as grades can be erroneously based on strength alone, they can also be based on so many items that a disproportionate amount of time is spent by each student and instructor on the task of grading. The grading chart improves organization and helps conserve grading time. A summary of our grading plan is shown in the chart below.

| | Skill and Performance 60% | | | | | Knowledge 20% | Social 20% | |
Name	Strength and Fitness	Skill	Im-prove-ment	Average	Weighted Scores	Knowl-edge	Social	Average
J. Doe	3	5	4	4	444	2	2	3

CODE: A......... 5   B......... 4   C......... 3   D......... 2   E......... 1

Figure 76. Grading Card for Weight Training

INDEX